I0807468

IT NEARLY KILLED ME

(But I Love You)

IT NEARLY KILLED ME

(But I Love You)

SINEAD CORCORAN DYE

A portrait of contemporary motherhood

MOA
PRESS

Published in New Zealand and Australia in 2025 by Moa Press
(an imprint of Hachette Aotearoa New Zealand Limited)
Level 2, 23 O'Connell Street, Auckland, New Zealand
www.hachette.co.nz
www.moapress.co.nz

Copyright © Sinead Corcoran Dye 2025

The moral right of Sinead Corcoran Dye to be identified as the author of this work has been asserted in accordance with the Copyright, Designs and Patents Act 1988.

All rights reserved. No part of this publication may be reproduced, stored in a retrieval system, or transmitted in any form or by any means, electronic, mechanical, photocopying, recording, or otherwise, without the prior permission of both the copyright owner and the above publisher of this book.

A catalogue record for this book is available from the National Library of New Zealand.

ISBN: 978 1 86971 833 6 (paperback)

Typeset by Cat Taylor in Minion Pro 11.6/15.3pt
Author photo by Kirsty Stone
Cover design by Cat Taylor and Meisha Kimber
Cover photo by Kirsty Stone
Printed and bound in Australia by McPherson's Printing Group

FSC www.fsc.org MIX Paper from responsible sources FSC® C001695

The paper this book is printed on is certified against the Forest Stewardship Council® Standards. McPherson's Printing Group holds FSC® chain of custody certification SA-COC-005379. FSC® promotes environmentally responsible, socially beneficial and economically viable management of the world's forests.

Hey pal,

Been thinking about you and how (fab a lot of the time of course!! But also) very fuckaroo this gig has turned out to be.

And I know usually people drop lasagnes etc. off when someone has a new baby or they're going through a (so so good of course!! But also) really hard time – but I do not know how to cook lasagne, nor any of the etcs.

So, we made you this instead. Hope some days it helps.

All our love,
Sinead, Michele & Vivie Michele
x

Contents

Introduction 1

Sunrise 5

Cluck cluck motherfucker 7

Positive role model? 11

I'm leaving you for McDreamy, bye 25

I don't remember 31

I remember 37

I don't want to go to Birthcare, I want to go to the clubs 45

If Breast Is Best then why do I hate her? 52

A week in the clink: what it's like to be hospitalised with PND 59

How he met your mother 71

My wonderful wife is cursed, by Stuart Dye 75

She hasn't died yet, but she will soon 85

Oh, OK so I'm raising Hell! 93

The lucky ones 103

I am Bono Corcoran Dye 110

3 a.m. secrets I will never tell your dad 115

Wanking at Baby Sensory class 119

Apps you need and apps you must delete 125

A sad beige baby 129

What you actually need to buy when you're having a baby. (This is the only list that matters.) 137

That's a shame 141

Sunset 149

My last will and testament 151

In the wrong hands 157

The Vivfluencer 161

3 a.m. maternity leave Google searches 167

Rate the pain from one to ten 171

3 a.m. *Dragons' Den* invention ideas 175

Guilty as sin 176

A tiny, curated selection of all the things I feel guilty about 185

A picture book for Vivie 189

Do we want to get divorced or do we just have young children? 196

When the weather turned 211

You've got a match! 221

Living the dream 230

I don't want to rule the world 251

Dear Sinead, I'm back baybay! 265

Acknowledgements 274

Endnotes 282

Introduction

I'D LIKE TO TELL YOU ABOUT A VERY GOOD DAY.

And no, it wasn't the day I gave birth and met my first child. That day was foul.

And the nine months of days leading up to that day were possibly the foulest days that have ever existed – definitely in my lifetime, but maybe actually the whole lifetime of the whole of humankind.

Oh, but the first two weeks of days after I had her, the dreamy, can't-believe-she's-here-and-she's-mine, soaking-up-every-snuggle, newborn-baby-bubble bliss?

Yeah, no – sorry. My newborn and I were shipped off in a paddy wagon (not really) to the clink (Starship Hospital's Mother & Baby Unit for cuckoo new mums).

Auckland's Penitentiary for Cuckoos is a specialised care unit with only three beds for three lucky mums who have the three most severe cases of postnatal psychiatric disorders in the country. And what you will soon learn is if there is a three in one zillion chance of something happening to someone, it will happen to me. Every time, guaranteed, *I* am the winner of the foulest lotto. But I like to think that this is actually me doing a good deed for humanity, like the 1News Good Sorts awards. Because if I take the hit then surely it means someone out there ducks under the punch coming their way – 'cause it's slammed me down instead. And on this occasion, it slammed me right into the slammer with this random stranger baby in tow.

But I shan't be telling you all the fascinating and grim details about life in lock-up right here in the introduction. Because if you've picked this book up maybe you're an absolute snake like me, AKA the kind of person who stands by the shelf reading the first couple of pages and then six hours later you're still standing there trying to finish the book to save yourself coughing up $39.99.

Anyway, back to when I (finally?) had A Very Good Day. It's coming. Not yet, but soon.

So, after I was finally released from clinky linky on good behaviour and returned home, I did what I aways do to get the sad and the pain and the trauma out of my head. Like, I drink a bit obvs, but I also do something productive. Something that might help someone else who's got sad and pain and trauma in them too.

I write.

And that day I wrote an essay on what it's like to stay in the clinky linky.

I wrote about what the past nine months had done to me and done to any chance I'd had at bonding with my brand-new daughter, my first child.

How those nine months nearly killed me. How, sometimes, I wished they had.

Because for a lot of that first year I knew without a shadow of a doubt that I must not be cut out to be a mum, especially to this baby who did not seem to belong to me. There must have been some mix-up at the fertility clinic – maybe all the Tupperware that houses the embryos fell on the floor and got jumbled like a lolly scramble? Because I certainly did not love her – I felt nothing towards her.

So, I wrote every dark thought, every intrusive thought I'd been having that I'd felt too ashamed to tell anyone. I wrote, I wrote, I wrote. I purged the poison onto pages.

And then I did what I always do – I gave it to a newspaper to run as a feature for a couple hundred bucks.

But when my editor came back, utterly traumatised from reading it, she said the piece was way too long to publish as is so she'd need to chop big chunks out and could only run part of it (just some scraps! The little shreds of chicken left on a gnawed-upon Wicked Wing!).

Some weird, Tony-Robbins-motivational-speaker voice inside me piped up at this and said 'Hey, this essay you've done. It's actually good. Like, really good. And it shouldn't be Wicked Wing shreds, it's bigger and better than that.'

So, I did what I've never done before – I said, *actually, thanks but no thanks.*

And then I did what I do occasionally (often) – I drank a bottle of red wine, got a bit ziggy, got a bit zaggy. Decided I am perhaps not just the most important voice of my generation but also the Queen Mother of all the mothers in the land? And I sent that story off to a big fancy book publisher instead.

And then the next day the publisher phoned to ask for a meeting.

They'd never had an entire office full of people crying after reading a pitch. They wanted to help make this book, which might help so many people, so many mums.

A week later my contract landed – a fancy stack of papers with a fancy publishing house logo on it, and my name. And I signed it.

And that was The Very Good Day.

A *quite proud of myself* day.

I called my best friends. They were quite proud of me too. But after getting off the phone with each of them I didn't feel right. I kept feeling like I had another call to make. I scrolled through my phone looking for the right person to tell. I had 'one celebratory drink' while I waited for my husband, Stu, to come home. I chewed all my nails off.

By the time he got in, I had drunk a bottle of wine. Because about three nails and three drinks in I realised that I was looking for my mum's number. Just like I did after my first date with him, and the day we got engaged, the day I found out I was pregnant, and as soon as I woke up after my C-section and became a mum too.

It's been nearly ten years since she died, so someone else has her number now. I know that because I accidentally called it, forgetting, when I got my first journalism job two weeks after she died. And I think that's why I write. I tell everyone everything because I want to tell my mum, but I can't.

Somewhere along the way this oversharing of my life, especially the hard stuff, seems to have helped people – women in particular. Mums in particular. And at thirty-two with a fresh newborn, I got a book deal because another mum, a big boss at a big publishing house, believed in me and my work and thought it could help even more women and mums.

This book is the biggest thing of my career, and my mum isn't here to see it.

So, instead, this book is for, and about, her.

It is for mums and stepmums and mums with mental illnesses and mums without mums.

This book is for me.

It represents hundreds of hours of writing, away from my baby – but that's okay because I still want to be Someone as well as being Mum, and I'm lucky that my work means helping others.

This book is for, and about, my daughter, Vivie.

It will remind me how cool it might feel for her one day to say her mum is an author.

One day I hope she reads it. One day I hope she even likes it.

I hope you will too.

Sunrise

@sineadcorcoran.dye
Stepmum, trophy wife, writer.
330 posts
5,588 followers
1,169 following

1 AUGUST 2023

Meet Genevieve Michele Dye – but Vivie to her pals (that's all of you!) <3

The last day of my nightmare, the first day of my forever girl

16 AUGUST 2021, 10:42 A.M.

Sinead: Fuck my life, man, we just went to the fertility clinic, and I said to the doctor:

'Hey before I ask you something on the sly, you just work here right, like on a salary? You don't own this place? And you don't get paid per customer, right? Just cause wouldn't want you to miss out on the money you'd get from our appointments. But do you reckon me and Stu could just do the turkey baster thing in our kitchen or whatever instead of proper IVF, because that would be free?'

And he said no because Stu's sperm is so shit they would just trickle back out, I guess.

Omg – like after sex when you're waiting for the guy to bring you a towel and you just lie there, frozen, like you've been shot? Like Squid Games?

And then you have to make like a rugby plastic crotch cup thing but it's your hand, and penguin waddle – but also somehow make it a sprint? – to the bathroom, all the while these tiny children are dripping out and you're like 'aww is this a bit sad maybe? I am their mum?'

It's those scenes but like, festive, because it's a turkey?

So anyway, I have to do the actual injections. And Stu won't do them for me since he can't even have a blood test because of his 'phobia of moving fluids'...???

Annabel: But he literally has to get a blood test as part of the IVF process! Also, another quite critical part of IVF relies on him moving some fluids into a cup?

Sinead: Yeah, he'll just die, I guess. That shall be the day he dies. And look, that's fine, I was raised by a single mum and I'm all good. Anyway, he was going to die one of these days and it had to be from something, ya know.

Cluck cluck motherfucker

LIKE HAVING A PARENT DIE YOUNG and becoming a stepmum at 27, IVF was another thing I was one of the first of my friends to go through.

I'd left my job shortly after Stu and I got engaged – not to be a lady of leisure, but because my dissociative disorder had become so severe I was unable to work in an office environment. Leaving work one day after a particularly bad episode, I crashed my car, and that's when we knew something had to give.

As I was unemployed for the foreseeable, we decided to take advantage of the time free of work commitments to undergo the first phase of IVF. We planned to freeze the embryos until after our wedding. We had tried for a year or two to get pregnant naturally, but we knew it wasn't likely as Stu had to do IVF for his sons, due to his low sperm motility.

There were some emotional complexities around this decision, as there always are when it comes to fertility challenges. I did feel guilty for pushing Stu to have a baby when he already had two kids, but having children together was something we'd discussed very early on. I also felt guilty that I was making him have a baby in his late forties, when all his other dad friends were coming out the other side of nappies and sleepless nights and finally getting their lives back.

But not guilty enough to not do it.

Besides, he'd made the choice to shack up with a woman in her twenties who was clear about wanting multiple children – and it was time to pay the piper.

I know by this point in the book – because you're a normal person who needs somewhat of a visual to care one iota about the people you are reading about – you have Googled.

And when you Googled me there was simply too much of a good thing, wasn't there? Approximately one million incredible pieces of my breathtaking hot takes but still not enough to satiate you for long – so you closed the tabs, vowing to only read one of my historic columns per year to savour them for as long as possible until your dying day where the final one would be read as your eulogy.

And you also had to close all the breathtaking Googy image tabs, because there simply weren't enough, were there? After the 2020 lockdown, my mental-health demise, then my IVF #journey, there were to be no more breaths taken. The woman who somewhat resembled quite-sexy Billie Piper was gone – and from then on was a mousey-haired Zorb, and you'd seen everything you needed to see, thanks.

So, then we moved on to Stu, didn't we? The elusive Stulusive.

And there is fuck all to stalk, I know. Trust me, I know. While Stu will have you believe it's because he's a prim and proper English gentleman who likes to keep his private life private and – unlike some very very sad people/Zorbs – does not require validation and praise from strangers on the internet in order to have the will to carry on, this is true … but this is not the whole truth.

The second half of that truth is that he does not exist on the worldwide web because I scrubbed him off it. Because even the tiny scraps of content he had posted online were never funny and his clothes were not good, and his hair was very bad, and it was, quite frankly, brand damaging.

So, on the eighth day of our courtship, I took his phone to the bathroom and delete, delete, delete. And so long Stu – We Hardly Knew Ye!

I did, however, generously allow him to retain a whole three images on the web, but this was solely for LinkedIn purposes as I must eat etc. So, I know that you know.

And it's okay, you can ask. I do not mind. I know you want to know why I married a little old papa.

I know you also know it is of course because of the issues. Of the papa variety. And far be it for me to disagree with this theory – if it looks like a duck/dad and your dad is a quack then it likely is daddy duck issues etc.

But it isn't just a duck that led me to a Dye. It was but a Dyery.

MESSAGE FROM DRIVER
(SINEAD CD, PRIUS DELOREAN, 0 STARS):

I have arrived.

Positive role model?

AND WHERE WE'RE GOING, WE DON'T NEED ROADS. Cause it's Friday Night and we're going to EZY Street baby.

In the noughties, the difference between a Good Friday Night and a Shit One depended on if your parent was fiscally responsible and had even a toddler-level grasp of maths – or if they were a yo-fucking-lo-er. Could they be convinced that the $8 Overnight New Release was better value than the 'Five Weeklies for $5' deal? Were they the regular Shit kind, or were they the Cool anti-vaxxers of their time – who eschewed movie classification labels and took M (suitable for mature audiences 16 years and over) as 'M-OST Likely Fine For Nine I Reckon'?

My mum was fucking cool.

So, on the Friday nights I went to a friend's house for a sleepover, we'd watch stuff like Chad Michael Murray bravely falls in love with very beautiful woman even though she works in a diner after school, basketball star Zac Efron agrees to overlook fellow classmate being intelligent and brunette and dates her nonetheless, etc.

And we of course watched *The Princess Diaries* – a beloved

chick flick that has stood the test of time and communicates many a powerful and important message to its fan base of little girls. Messages like, how to be brave and stand up to bullies - and that change doesn't mean losing yourself, it means finding yourself in the process, even when it seems scary.

For me personally, every watch was a mixed bag, as every viewing also reconfirmed the notion that if you straighten your hair and take your glasses off you will be hot now - but I VS Sassooned my side fringe approximately thrice daily and I didn't wear glasses thus they have always and will always be off? AKA ... is this my final form? Is this as good as it gets?

And what was almost as deflating - as I'm sure it was for daughters of single mums everywhere - was when our mums had to say 'so sorry to - for the ninth time - be the confirmer of bad news, but yes to the best of my knowledge I have not fucked a rich prince and the peasant man you know to be your father is sadly your real father'.

But the nights I stayed home with my mum, it was *Bridget Jones's Diary*.

As I write this, I have just looked up the parental ratings and the reviews written by parents themselves. My favourite is inserted below, which I hereby in this para give written consent for my publisher to use as my posthumous author bio if for some reason I perish before this book is released.

Positive role model?
Bridget makes a lot of foolish mistakes, smokes a lot and drinks when she's depressed. Proceed with caution.[1]

I thank my lucky stars everyday that Michele threw caution to the Dunhill Blue-fumed wind, because together, Renée Zellweger & my mum instilled into me over and over again that when it comes to men, the sky's the fucking limit, baby. Even if you don't have Anne Hathaway's big Bambi eyes (and actually your eyes are so curiously small that, like Renée's, they are barely visible to the human eye) all is not lost when it comes to finding love, my friend.

Bridget Jones's Diary and my mother told me that there is in fact a very, very, very small – so small it's barely visible to the human eye – catchment of hot, upper-class, highly educated, well-mannered, very emotionally repressed but also very kind British men who might possibly be open to maybe considering entertaining the idea of dating a very fat (size 10) normal-looking person.

And that man will like you just as you are. Which is not even just that you maybe work in a diner or, even more challenging to overcome, you're brunette. He actually will tolerate that you're a fucking nuthead.

So yes, I likely was drawn to the papas because Call Me Big Papa Issues.

But I believe it might also be more complex – that my papareferences, if you will, may have also been influenced and reinforced by the media I was exposed to that starred a very specific type of male figure. Not the young hot ones like Chad Michael Murray, but the boring, reliable, kind dad-types. And that these two factors – no papa, sí papá on TV – they butterfly-effected me right to who I said I Do to.

My mum and I watched Bridget Jones so many times. And during those last few watches, towards the end, I was in my early twenties – so I was old enough for the 'lessons to be learned' to be padded out with crucial detail.

For years both Bridget and my mother had taught me that it's absolutely critical to marry a reliable, kind man. And that actually when you're a fucking nuthead, boring men are a very sensible choice because they will keep you tethered firmly and safely to the ground when you're being said nuthead.

Then, towards the end, my mum told me there would only ever be one thing I could ever do that would make her so disappointed. And that would be if, right out the gate, I married and settled down with a reliable, kind, boring Mark Darcy and was shacked up with kids in my twenties, before I'd even lived.

That there was so much time to find my Mark Darcy and do all that living – that your twenties are for fun, and fun is fucking all the Daniel Cleavers.

That if one day she peeped her head up from the blazing flames of hell where she will of course be residing, and I was half of one of those deeply sad, married 23-year-old Christian couples who move to Tauranga for a 'quieter pace of life' – instead of having many threesomes with many Daniel Cleavers – she would be so, so angry with me.

And we cannot have that!

But I must fast-forward through those Golden Years because my father-in-law is a retired Methodist minister, and I love him very much. It is very likely that he won't even make it this far because he may drop dead when he trots past a Whitcoulls and sees this book on the shelf. Even now, while I'm still writing it, we believe he thinks I am printing out 'Some Blogs,' stapling them together and selling them 'On the Blogs'.

If he has not yet passed on to the next realm, I cannot risk killing him with my tales of my Golden Years, because far be it for me to let down my dead mum!

After making really, really, really sure my mum would not be devastated, I did marry a Darcy. And not just one who generously likes me just as I am. And not just because he also keeps me tethered firmly and safely to the ground when I'm blasting off. But because he's like, 'okay you fucking freak, I see you! And I am very very uncomfortable with what I see! But yo-fucking-lo I will relocate to Freak Town and now it's population: 2!' And he's so scared and he can't stop crying.

At time of writing, we have been together nearly six years, and we probably only have six left at best, because he is like one of those shaking and spindly little retired greyhounds and not even a turtleneck will be enough to protect him against the vicious and unrelenting elements of Freak Town. So, in the interest of spending as much quality time as we can together and keeping him comfortable at home, I cannot waste these precious moments telling you everything divine about him. Just know he is nearly perfect except that he lives in my home and is the father of my children, so I must interact with him regularly which nearly kills me, but I love him so much. And just to retain one iota of your care about the people in this book – here is a very small glimpse at how dedicated he is to upholding his permanent residency in Freak Town.

When, very early on in our courtship, I once asked him if he'd like to play Hide & Seek, he was the only man who has ever not assumed I was referring to some form of sex game. He knew that what I was referring to was the Hiding & the Seeking game. And he said yes to the Hiding & the Seeking. And when it came time for his turn to hide, that man did not fuck around. He was not here to play games, oh no. He knew no entry-level amateur spot like some half-assed behind-the-curtain crap would prove he was the true man I had been seeking for so long.

So that man fucking MANNE FRANKED.

I spent two hours ransacking our apartment to no avail, and this apartment was the size of a toasted sandwich. But this man is no bigger than a peanut.

I continued to search. I screamed his name. I beseeched and I bescreeched for this tiny grain of sand. It was quite literally like searching for a needle in a haystack. He would later explain how he had hidden INSIDE the kids' bunk beds. Not under the duvet, inside the literal bunk scaffolding. This man Andy Dufresne'd his way in by somehow prising open some slats and slithering in like the rat he is.

One time he asked if I wanted a massage, and I said OK, and he was the only man who did not then proceed to give me two friendly pats on the back before commencing doggy-style. Instead, when I said OK, I was provided the address for East Dye Spa, which was our address. And upon arriving at the spa, which was our living room,

I was greeted with candlelight and the tranquil sound of groaning dementors, which was apparently a sound-bath playlist. And when the mobile masseuse arrived, they bowed to me and they were also Ma Stuse. And he was wearing a little white dress.

I didn't know why. I said 'Why?' and he said 'What? This is what they wear?' and I said 'What? Where have you been for massages?' and he said nothing for a very long time, which has been six years now.

One night when Vivie was about three weeks old, I announced 'Right, enough is enough'. I told Stu to 'wake the fuck up' and realise we had been revolving our sad little lives around this baby for far too long, while our marriage had fallen by the wayside – that I couldn't believe I hadn't seen the signs sooner – and that it was vital that we prioritise regularly watering the plant that is our love with a minimum of twice-weekly date nights to Bring Back The Spark.

He said OK but suggested perhaps we start with at-home date nights seeing as our daughter was still unvaccinated thus should probably not be carted out to SPQR, and also I might be more comfortable at home as my C-section was still basically in two flesh sections 'and also a week ago you were basically sectioned?'.

So I said OK. But I also said 'well guess what Stu, if you think a half-assed "at-home date night" means half an episode of *Only Murders in the Building* then clearly we're on really different pages when it comes to the sanctity of marriage and by that I mean I think what we're looking at here is Irreconcilable Differences'. He said OK. And when it came his turn to host date night I arrived home to Only Murders in Our House.

'Oh Inspector, thank goodness you're here – I have a most baffling case for you!' he cried.

My dining room table was covered in a splay of 'evidence' like 'police reports' and 'suspect mugshots' and every single one of the suspects was an out-of-work, former Shortland Street actor. And I felt so very sad knowing they were surely paid $30 at most for signing their likenesses away to this sad little board game.

There behind the table - grey-haired, bespectacled and wrapped in a knitted shawl - sat the littlest little old lady the world has ever known. He was wearing a name tag that said Mrs Markle. (If you want to see documentation of this, I urge you to go look at my Instagram. It was both widely appalling but also very well received.) Months after we did not solve the case - because it was actually really hard and I just could not get invested when each suspect was someone who is now a sad little real estate agent – I asked Stu 'Hey what the fuck re that costume?' and he said 'What do you mean?'

I said 'She doesn't look anything like that?' and he said 'What do you mean?' before we established that while he was wearing a Miss Marple costume, I thought he meant social worker, former makeup artist and yoga instructor Doria Ragland, as in, mother of Meghan.

And now you know why I love him so much, because he will do the most fucked-up shit to make me happy, and Vivie darling that's how babies are made. <3

Because Stu fancied himself a nice 'n' easy little dinner, didn't he? A little rotiss spring chicken from Countdown & a couple of baps? Well, that chicken came home to roost and guess who the sweaty bag of meat was then? And I felt like Chicken Tonight and it was Stu on the menu, how divine! And there was nowhere to run and there was nowhere to hide because when that bug-eyed and scattery Chicken Little looked around him it was nothin' but net. Because he was not home on the range, no siree - he was a caged battery hen. And it was time to lay in the bed he made.

I'd tell him that lots of celebrities have kids older, like Al Pacino and Robert De Niro, and he'd counter that these people are incredibly wealthy and can afford round-the-clock childcare, which surely makes a difference. At our first IVF consultation we discovered that we didn't qualify for public funding, because Stu had already had two children through IVF, even though he had gone private. I was furious. I thought I should be entitled to access the public system to have my own biological children – particularly as Stu hadn't even used public funding. Stu assured me that even if we did qualify, going through the public system can often take a couple of years, so we would have gone private anyway. A couple of years isn't really so small when anything can happen in a couple of years. My mum was a runner, and she ate so much salad and had regular appointments with a chiropractor. She flossed her teeth everyday - not just like a normal person who does it once a year before seeing the dentist so you can truthfully say 'yes I do floss'. And when she was the same age as Stu is now, they told her she was down to her last couple of years, and that the best ones were definitely behind her.

So, I refused to wait a 'couple of years' when I was attempting to have a child with a man who hadn't frequented a GP since he left Britain 16 years prior, and also still abided by the apparent British cultural norm of drinking one single cup of water per fortnight. This is a man whose urine is surely the colour of Lipton Iced Tea. Our child was going to need all the couples they could get.

We forked out a fortune for the process, and I began injections.

My high-school friend Annabel, the only person I knew who had gone through IVF, was my absolute rock through the process – even sitting with me on FaceTime for my first injection. Stu has the worst fear of needles I've ever encountered (he nearly passes out at a simple blood test), so I had to inject myself, though I made him watch. I thought he deserved it after all I was having to go through while he just had to masturbate into a cup. So mean right? Or – so smart?

When Stu reads this, he will finally learn the truth, that the injections didn't even hurt LOL! And shame because he bought me a Cricut to say sorry.

I did however spend my days vomiting in the sink – an omen for my pregnancy to come. And then came the pessaries – huge tablets you have to insert three times a day, to the minute – which meant I'd have to run to the bathroom halfway through a movie or dinner out. Disgustingly dubbed 'fanny lollies' on fertility forums, they were itchy and leaked out into my underwear.

I resented Stu through the process. He was the one with low motility sperm; he was the reason that we didn't qualify for public funding; he was the reason I was vomiting in the sink. It didn't seem fair. But then, the physical and emotional toll on the person carrying the baby rarely is.

When it came time for the egg retrieval, I was so swollen and had been in so much pain during my internal exams that we paid another chunk of money for me to be put under for the procedure – another omen. And then we paid more to have Stu's sperm injected into the eggs because they wouldn't swim in there themselves. More resentment.

I knew this resentment was utterly unfair, too – fertility issues are no one's 'fault' – but it simmered away nonetheless. I wasn't in therapy at the time, which is where, historically, I vented about my deep, dark, unfair thoughts, and Annabel's Polycystic ovary syndrome (PCOS) was the 'reason' her and her partner had to do fertility treatment, so I definitely couldn't vent to her. Which meant that, as I had nowhere to let the steam of resentment out, the simmering turned into bubbling and sometimes bubbled right over – scalding Stu. Notable mentions include the two occasions he made the dire mistake of existing, and I deleted and blocked him on Facebook.

The successful embryos were frozen, and I cried my eyes out on the drive home. Jacked up on hormones, I felt devastated that I was abandoning my 'children' alone in a freezer. I thought about fashioning them natty little knits to wear and if I could ask to put a UE Boom in the tank and play them Taylor Swift in the hopes it would somehow Animorph them into the girls I was desperate for so I could recreate the Gilmore Girls-esque bond I had with my mum. We already had two boys at home, and two is company and three is a crowd and two is also a crowd when you're talking about young boys.

Now – to avoid as much hate mail as possible – I must preface what I'm about to say next with three statements. The first is, I am utterly grateful to have been in a position where we could afford to pay for IVF – a luxury devastatingly not accessible to many families. The second is, aside from my husband being one very dehydrated foot in the grave, we also had the luxury of choosing when to do said IVF, on the basis/hope it would be straightforward and quick to work as I didn't have any apparent fertility issues. The third is, every body is beautiful etc, we are all a Dove campaign, real women have curves, slim women I guess are not real and maybe ghosts.

Okay and just now while writing this I had a repressed memory emerge from the recesses of my mind. Remember Trinny and Susannah? And where the fuck are they now and why isn't it jail?

If you are reading this, I assume you are a person who was born in the same millennium as me, which means I am certain you know if you are an Apple or a Pear, or a body shape dubbed something even more devastating - The Brick. But if you are reading this from the future (thank you for the continuous royalties as I have no money to pass down to Vivie, only many mental-health issues) - fucking buckle up because you don't even know how lucky you are to be blithely unaware that you have 'chicken wing arms', 'thunder thighs' and/or 'tits like fried eggs'.

The basic premise of the show *What Not To Wear* was that two women - Skinny Trinny and Regular-Sized Susannah - would find someone who was going about their life perfectly fine and of relatively sound mind and spirit, and say the equivalent of 'Hey! You are actually repulsive!' They would proceed with a filmed autopsy where they would thoroughly examine said person and offer helpful assessment notes such as 'she's very top-heavy' and 'from the waist up you're an old frump'. Most notable moments of the series include participants being obliterated so violently they collapsed wailing, and that time Susannah once spontaneously pulled someone's underwear down during filming as her 'knicker line was visible' and we all nodded and said, 'yup, only fair'.

The next stage involved rotating the now emotionally decimated husk like a donor kebab before a 360-degree mirror while Trinny and Susannah dissected her appearance from the front, the back and the side and probably inside too. Then, after a fun shopping spree where the kebab was guided on choosing the right clothes to cloak her meat in, came a selection of my favourite takeaway tips:

'Decoration on the body will help detract attention from your hefty legs.'

'Thin straps only highlight the enormity of your upper arms.'

'Don't wear a belted coat because it increases the width of your uncontrollable girth.'[2]

Yes, of course every body is beautiful – chicken, lamb and mixed etc. But could one of these beautiful bodies maybe have let me know that if you do IVF just a few short months before your wedding, you do run the risk of becoming the exact same girth as the Earth?

Which is absolutely fine, of course. I have always and will likely always be a curvy person, and I am very lucky that this is now the trending cut of meat. I am just saying, a heads up would have been nice so that I was prepared to gain thirty kilograms in about thirty minutes, and then for my (strangely) relatively unchanged body to be a mere guest at my own wedding – while my thirty-kilogram face Zorbed down the aisle.

A week after our wedding, I Zorbed right back into Fertility Associates and we had the first embryo implanted. Stu warned me that first IVF attempts often don't work, but that second ones do as your body is more prepped for a baby. I don't know why I trusted this, as he's no medical expert – remember, this man hasn't been to the GP in sixteen years – but I believed him and prepared for the worst.

We had to wait ten days from implantation to find out if it had worked. I tried to put the whole thing out of my mind and lasted until day eight before breaking down in my car and calling Annabel, bawling and wracked with anxiety. On day nine I couldn't wait anymore. I had a job interview that afternoon but could barely concentrate on preparing – my mind was so preoccupied with getting the results. Despite being told not to do a home test (as it can give a false result), I drove to get KFC and accidentally-on-purpose picked up a test while out.

I peed on the stick and ate Wicked Wings while I waited.

Two lines appeared during the second wing.

My first call was not to my husband, but to Annabel, tentatively elated. I then phoned Stu – he was excited but warned me that we needed to wait for the blood test the next day.

I desperately wanted a glass of wine to celebrate but restrained myself.

An hour later, I did not pay attention as the interviewers asked me questions, and I gave them pathetic, unenthused answers. But it didn't matter because I was maybe, hopefully, having a baby! (Unsurprisingly, they did not offer me the job.)

The next day the clinic phoned while we were driving, and I got Stu to film the phone call with the idea of posting a heart-warming video when – if – we made the announcement. But again, as I am incredibly, incredibly lucky to so far have not had any fertility issues – I truly was nowhere near the edge of my seat.

Because on the 5th and the 12th of February 2006,[3] when Christina Ricci's character on *Grey's Anatomy* fucking see-ya-ed her hand right out of that man's stomach and Meredith punched her hand in to catch the bomb and then Kyle Chandler tippy-toed it down the hall and we all took one single breath, nothing can scare me anymore. And even though we were all like 'Kyle We Hardly Knew Ye!' when he and his little vest got blown to smithereens, our nervous systems were also what military historians would go on to definitively classify as Perpetually Fucked. And when recent studies declared millennials the most anxious generation in history, it is because we have all been shallow panting and gasping for oxygen since February 2006. So, 'Congratulations, you're pregnant'?

Nice!

11 JANUARY 2023, 6:47 P.M.

Sinead: Sin is in the worst season of her life

Sinead: The only thing keeping me from ending it all is that once every six weeks I get to see my OB. This is simply all I have to live for.

Harry: Who is he?

Sinead: [name redacted]

Sinead: *image*

Harry: Omg he's gorgeous

Sinead: He is BDE ay

Harry: Is he a gay man?

Sinead: Married to a woman – confusing that I am not this woman

Sinead: At our last appt when he pulled down my pants to do a scan I was significantly aroused

Harry: Are we going to sleep with our obstetrician?

Harry: We are ay

Sinead: Yup

Harry: Extraordinary

I'm leaving you for McDreamy, bye

STU DIDN'T CRACK WHILE HURTLING AROUND the lampless dirt roads of rural Auckland and slithering through the throngs of Warriors fans at small-town RSAs to get to the tucked-away freezer. His exhausted and petrified frozen claws pawed through expired Trumpets to find the last remaining Grapefruit Frujus in the land. Because the one single food that his sick wife didn't vomit up had recently been discontinued by Tip Top, sparking a nationwide outrage that made headlines, even among those who weren't violently ill.

'To her, the ice blocks were far more than just a summer nice-to-have – over the last few months they had been an edible lifeline.

'"When I received the news today from Tip Top confirming they have been discontinued, I burst into tears," says Grapefruit Fruju devotee Sinead Corcoran Dye.

'It was around a month ago that she last found the ice block, at a dairy in the West Auckland suburb of Henderson ... "Had I known it would be the last time, I would have treasured every lick. I would have bought 15 of them.'"[4]

Stu didn't crack when I, upon learning he had planned nothing for my 31st birthday, screamed 'IT'S NOT THAT FUCKING HARD!' in his frightened, pale face. The frightened, pale face of a man whose incredibly sick and incredibly volatile pregnant wife had previously given him strict instructions *not* to plan anything for her birthday because 'there's no fucking point when I can't drink!' He didn't crack when I then asked him 'why the fuck' he hadn't put a crumb of thought into coming up with a 'nice, pampery, sober' activity instead, 'like a high tea and massages at a hotel for me and a friend? Honestly it's, like, not that fucking hard, Stu.'

He didn't crack when, hands shaking while entering his credit card details, he paid a cold-sweat-inducing fortune for a last-minute 'BFF Staycation package' at a five-star hotel, which included:

- A stylish room
- Valet parking
- An exquisite high tea
- A delicious breakfast
- A spa pamper gift pack
- A heated rooftop pool and jacuzzi
- A herbal steam room and sauna
- A massage and a facial

Stu didn't crack when, upon my return home, he asked if I'd had a good time and I muttered, 'Well, don't know why the fuck you booked high tea, to be honest, when you know I hate high tea. I don't eat sweet stuff, hello? And wow what a birthday feast – cold, sad little sandwiches? Yeah cheers, thanks, best birthday ever.'

And he didn't even crack when, on the way home from our 30-week scan, I showed him the original floor plan sketches of our obstetrician's house that I had dug up from the depths of Google.

'Six bedrooms, see, and his children are teenagers, so they'll be moved out of home soon and there'll definitely be room for our baby and the babies we'll have together.'

By *together* I didn't mean my husband and I, I meant my husband-to-be – the man I would absolutely, no doubt in my mind, leave Stu for – my obstetrician. And look, it wasn't just me who had the horn. When I had bleeding early on in my pregnancy, I was admitted to hospital to monitor the baby. A nurse, upon finding out who my OB was, said, 'Lucky girl, we call him McDreamy.' Enough said.

I spent my second trimester deep-diving the internet, not only repeatedly reading the one news article he'd ever featured in and every study or medical journal he'd ever contributed to, but everything his wife had ever featured in too. I knew her maiden name and the primary school she went to.

'She's not even that pretty?' I'd scoff at Stu. He'd nod in agreement.

But she was pretty.

At 34 weeks pregnant I woke up and told my husband I'd had a dream that our OB and his wife had invited us over to have group sex. Stu asked how it went. I told him I'd actually gone alone; I hadn't extended the invitation to him but, yes, it was great. He patted my hand, nodded and said, 'Well, that's good.'

At 36 weeks pregnant, when I was yet again hospitalised with dehydration and hooked up to an IV, I managed to hunt down one of my OB's teenage sons' Instagram accounts and combed through every post trying to find a photo of his father, with a precision usually deployed for detonating bombs or that board game where you gingerly try to extract the body parts – except my operation was avoiding 'liking' any of the posts accidentally.

And despite spending every single day on the couch in mismatched pajamas, with a greasy bun and reeking of vomit, each appointment we had with him I would use what tiny shreds of strength I had to wash my hair, fake tan my face (at the very least) and put on my somewhat flattering Lululemon leggings. I'd douse myself (my crotch in particular, obviously) with the only expensive perfume I've ever owned – and only use on special occasions – Le Labo, which Stu had bought me.

At 38 weeks, a few days before I'd have my daughter, I was in hospital again on IVs and with straps around my belly that monitored her heart for dehydration and distress. I was very distressed about her potential distress. But I was also very distressed when my OB made a surprise visit to my room – an unexpected date!

As he checked mine and my daughter's vitals, I lay there furious that I was wearing sweaty pajamas. He perched on a chair eating an apple and making polite small talk with the sick, sad pregnant woman. But all the woman could think about was that she wished she was the apple.

But she would never be the apple. Because she stunk.

The night before my elective C-section, I made Stu shave my entire vagina because I knew our OB would see it. I was categorically insane.

And even then, hunched down on the floor shaving his pale, gaunt, nine-months pregnant wife's vagina to 'impress' another man, Stu never cracked.

I think he knew that this definitely unrequited crush was truly the only thing getting me through the nightmarish days. He understood that, like most mothers, I had deprived myself of anything that I usually rely on to regulate my emotions or bring me any sense of joy – whether that was food (couldn't keep any down), sex (we tried but Stu couldn't bring himself to put me through any physical exertion when I was so sick and withered), alcohol, nicotine, caffeine or socialising. Even my antidepressants and anti-anxiety medication had been taken away. I had nothing. All I had was frenetic wanking about my doctor. And look, I know you're probably thinking that someone should have called the cops, or at the very least had a quiet word with the good doctor about perhaps dropping me as a patient and filing a light restraining order – but I have googled this madness and it's not just me. Pregnant women all over everywhere are falling in love with their OBs.

In 1999, a pregnant woman wrote to *LA Times* advice columnist, Vicki.[5]

'How common is it for a woman to develop a crush on her obstetrician while she is pregnant? During my pregnancies, I would find myself constantly thinking about my doctor and comparing my husband to him. I noticed how cool and nice he was and how nice he probably was to his wife and kids. At the same time, I felt myself repulsed by my husband. Why was this happening? Strange pregnancy hormones?'

Vicki understood. 'By my third and fourth pregnancies, nothing could get me to shave my legs, blow dry my hair or change out of my overstretched and shiny leggings except my monthly visit to my obstetrician. I even put extra perfume between my ankles, since he seemed to spend much of his time down there. Somewhere near the beginning of each visit he would ask me how I was, and I would nearly weep with gratitude – he really seemed to care what my answer would be. It's natural to develop strong feelings for the one person you're convinced stands between you and the certain death that labor and delivery might otherwise bring. He's not just a man, he's Superman.'

Vicki understands. I understand. My husband understands. He allowed the many, many wanks. And that's how I know I should probably not leave him; he is a very good man.

Also, on the off-chance this book falls into my OB's hands, I am quite certain any shred of attraction he (most definitely did not) have for me may very likely turn into a touch of fear and alarm. And he will likely file that light restraining order.

And, look, fair enough.

1 AUGUST 2023, 10:15 A.M.

Sinead: A very hot nurse man came in and put heart monitors on my bare boobs

Sinead: He said do you want me to get a female chaperone and I said <3 no <3

Harry: AHAHHAHHA

Sinead: I'm scared Haz

Harry: Wot bout? C sec?

Sinead: Meeting my baby. What if she hates me?

Harry: Omg don't worry about that!

Harry: Of course she will!

Harry: We have known that since conception

Sinead: It was written in the stars ay

Harry: It was. And that will never change x

I don't remember

I'VE TRIED TO WRITE ABOUT MY PREGNANCY over and over again, but I don't remember being pregnant. All I remember is being sick, and even much of that has slipped away. Sometimes I say to Stu that I know I vomited a few times, but it wasn't that bad. It terrifies him when I say this, because he remembers it all.

Unable to keep food (and later, water) down, right up until my daughter's birth; countless hospitalisations on IVs for both my and her dehydration; rib flare (look it up – horrendous) and a broken foot (dropped a statue – another story); unable to get out of bed most days, let alone work; incontinence and adult nappies; damaged teeth. Stu remembers it *all*…

Someone once asked me how sick Sinead was, so one day I decided to count how many times she vomited. It was 22. That wasn't a particularly bad day, nor a comparatively good day. I'd say it was a normal day.

In between vomiting, she spent time sleeping, talking about how sick she felt or, occasionally, in a good moment, being swept up by false hope that perhaps the worst was over. She couldn't work or see friends; she could barely maintain a conversation about anything other than how sick she felt. Heartbreakingly, she became a stranger to the boys.

The strain on all of us was enormous. It was profoundly disruptive – we couldn't make plans, we had to cancel things for the boys, I became unreliable at work. These are all trivial when up against the monster of hyperemesis gravidarum (HG), but they are the pillars that shape and hold life together, and they were gone.

Then came the frequent hospital trips; hours spent hooked up to a drip for fluids and medication. Every second or third day. It was chaos – it hit us like an earthquake, shaking our steady ground and ripping new seams where we once stood. It devastated Sinead, and it was devastating to be a helpless bystander.

So, we adapted to a new reality. I thought Sinead just had to survive this sickness and we just had to cope until it passed. But HG – much like any long-term sickness, I guess – had another brutal trick up its sleeve. Being bedridden and hospitalised and vomiting 22 times a day took a mental toll on Sinead that was as bad as the physical symptoms.

If you visit someone with a newborn baby, their description of pregnancy or the pain of childbirth often includes the phrase 'never again,' and, according to Stu, I said that phrase every day of those nine long, pregnant months.

I don't remember that.

Those months are a blur of sleep and vomit and wanting to drink to numb it all – but not being allowed to.

Sleep, vomit, rinse and repeat.

The only time I remember how bad the pregnancy truly was nowadays is roughly once a month if I encounter a hyperemesis trigger food or drink. For me it's often meat, or lukewarm coffee, and it will make me vomit after just a bite or sip.

My friend, who is a nurse studying HG and its lasting trauma, believes there may be a physiological reason as to why I'm more sensitive to vomiting now; that perhaps it's because the sphincters within my esophagus are worn out from throwing up so much that, now, they struggle to keep the contents of my stomach in when I'm triggered.

According to the Hyperemesis Education and Research (HER) Foundation[6], recovery from HG, which affects less than two out of every 100 pregnant women, takes an average of four to six months – but may take a few years if the illness was severe or prolonged, like mine was: from a week after getting pregnant right up until Vivie was taken out of me.

Food aversions may take months or even years to overcome, and lasting side effects can include stomach, throat and tooth damage, stomach ulcers and bacterial imbalance, low bone density due to malnutrition, muscle atrophy, depression, anxiety or trauma. Tick, tick, tick.

In 2022, a mum in the UK a few years younger than me, called Jess Cronshaw, was suffering severe HG – and Jess and her partner felt her medical care team 'weren't listening to them.' At seven months pregnant and 'reduced to a shell', Jess killed herself.

Her baby was born by emergency C-section twelve weeks early but did not survive.

A coroner's inquest in January 2024 heard how the cumulative impact of failings in Jess's care resulted in a severe deterioration of her mental health, and that guidelines relating to HG were ambiguous.[7]

Despite the risks to women and their unborn children, HG is disgracefully under-researched. My OB once told me that if men suffered it, you could guarantee there would be a cure by now.

It was only at the end of 2023 that a study suggested there was hope of a cure. Scientists found babies produce a hormone that can cause severe sickness. They believe exposure to the GDF15 hormone ahead of pregnancy could be a new treatment. It surely can't be a coincidence that this research emerged after Kate Middleton suffered HG through her pregnancies.

Charlotte Howden, CEO of the UK charity Pregnancy Sickness

Support, which supports women with HG, said the health issue had been neglected for too long.

'I'm so grateful for the dedication of the researchers, because this isn't a condition that really ever made the headlines until the Princess of Wales suffered with it.

'It wasn't an area of research that people were really interested in. It was just morning sickness - why should we care?'[8]

What I do remember from my pregnancy is fighting through tears with our obstetrician for an early C-section, trying to convince him that I was at breaking point physically and mentally and that *that* needed to come before the small risk of Vivie needing a breathing tube.

I do remember the phone call on 31 July, telling us to come to the hospital first thing the next morning to be on standby for a slot – like we were off to the airport for a flight.

I do remember spending the day in a private room – because I couldn't stop vomiting in the waiting room – and being slumped on the bed, dry-retching into a paper cup, with a crippling migraine from dehydration.

I do remember, at 3:15 p.m., a nurse barrelling in saying that in 15 minutes I was going to have a daughter.

I don't remember waking up and being handed a baby, but it must have happened because there she was.

In an evolutionary sense, memory of pain serves an important purpose. It indicates a threat to our safety or our life, and human survival depends on us avoiding things that we already know are going to kill us. But somehow there's an exception to that rule.

The pain and the trauma of childbirth, for lots of women, even soon after birth, feels like a distant dream that *wasn't really that bad actually* – when in fact it was a nightmare. So we do it over and over again, maybe because if we remembered the pain of childbirth – and, in my case, a pregnancy that nearly killed me – women might never go back, and thereby threaten the survival of the species.

But the myth that women are biologically programmed to forget the pain of childbirth, or the trauma of an incredibly difficult pregnancy, is also fostered by the language we use to describe the euphoria and relief of delivering a healthy baby. At the moment of holding their child for the first time, women often report that the pain of labour has all but been forgotten. It hasn't really been forgotten, but the happiness and the reward colour the memory of the preceding pain. This is known as the halo effect.[9]

But I didn't get a halo.

Because I can't remember the birth, because I wasn't really there. I didn't actually show up in the end. I really did try – I promise I did, Vivie. But I'm not a runner and I was so tired I couldn't even make it to the finish line. Couldn't even make it to my own baby. I didn't deserve a reward, not even a participation award. And even if I did – I wasn't even there to get my prize. Someone else had to take it on my behalf.

So, I didn't get a halo. I didn't get to heaven. I thought I'd been through hell and back but turns out I wasn't being sent back after all. Instead, a layover – landing and locked up in purgatory.

I remember what happened next.

5 AUGUST 2023, 10:18 A.M.

Georgia: Hey, Chlo said you had to be put to sleep to have the baby?? Isn't that really rare?? What happened are you OK???

Sinead: Yeah, nothing happened I just fucked it all up Georg

I remember

I CAN'T REMEMBER THE BIRTH, but this is what I've been told.

I know when I was wheeled into the OR, I had a panic attack on the operating table, because Stu said that's what happened.

He said that I couldn't stop shaking in terror, but that it was much worse than that, and frightening to watch – that I was convulsing, like I was having a seizure. He said I told him my arms and legs felt like the bones were being snapped from the pain of them uncontrollably thrashing around.

He said they tried to put an epidural in three or four times, but it kept getting knocked around and knocked out because I couldn't stay still, couldn't stop seizing.

(An orthopaedist has since told me that these failed injections must have hit nerves in my spine when they were being knocked around. He said that's why, for the eight months after I gave birth, my left leg was numb from the knee down, with constant pins and needles in my foot, which made it difficult to sleep.)

Stu said I then told the doctors I needed to be given the strongest relaxing sedatives that they had, now.

He said the doctors told us the drugs would work by relaxing my body and mind, so we'd assumed some sort of high-strength clonazepam. Instead, when the drugs hit my bloodstream I started panicking even more. He said that I told him it was what I imagined having your drink spiked feels like. That I had tried to speak but to me it sounded like I was underwater. That I was terrified the doctors couldn't hear me saying I needed to be put under.

Stu said that I grabbed the collar of his shirt, wrenching him towards my face, petrified – like I was trying to scream a message urgently to him with my eyes and praying he understood. He said he took one look at me and barked at them to put me to sleep, now.

When I woke up from the general anaesthetic, I didn't ask to hold my baby. I didn't ask about her at all. Because when I first came to, I didn't remember the primary reason I had been put to sleep.

So, instead of asking to see my baby, the first words that came out of my mouth were panicked babbling, asking Stu if everyone was mad at me because I had been 'such a handful' on the operating table, and that I was so sorry I couldn't do it, and was he disappointed in me? He was, I knew it, I knew it, and I was so sorry, so sorry, I know I messed it all up.

Eventually Stu reminded me that a baby was here now, and would I like to meet her?

I don't remember saying yes. I was too busy apologising over and over again for doing it all wrong.

I have photos and a video of me holding Vivie after she was born, which I now know were taken quite a while after. In the video – in which I look utterly dazed and confused, but I suppose every new mum does – I have one single Meghan Markle-esque chic tear rolling down my cheek. Crying, like every mum does when they meet their child – overwhelmed with relief the birth is over, and overwhelmed with joy and love.

That's not why *I* was crying though.

I was crying because I had been too scared and too weak to have a proper C-section and see my baby be born.

And maybe I would have shaken that all off and been able to reassure myself that very few births go to plan; that I did the right thing by going to sleep and not putting myself through any more fear and trauma, so that I was in the best possible shape for when the baby arrived; that all that mattered was she was here now and she was perfectly okay and healthy; and, of course, no one was mad at me for any of it.

Except I didn't shake it off.

When we arrived at Birthcare and one of the doctors who had been in the operating room arrived, I started apologising profusely again, saying I'm so sorry I made them have a shit afternoon at work, and I know it wasn't ideal and I should have done better and been braver.

I didn't shake it off, because the doctor didn't reassure me that very few births go to plan, that I made the right choice in the circumstances. The doctor's response was, 'Yeah look, I'll be honest. You did okay. But you didn't do great.'

A week later, everyone was so baffled as to why this new first-time mum wasn't bonding with her baby, and *what on Earth were the chances that after she was smacked down with HG for nine months, she also develops postnatal depression?*

And it was all so confusing because, according to the medical records, the operation had gone smoothly; the baby was perfectly okay and healthy.

But there are no medical records for what happened when I woke up. No record stating that this first-time mum didn't ask to hold her baby – didn't even remember there was a baby. Because I was convinced I had failed at motherhood before I'd even begun, so I knew I would fail at everything that was to come next. And this belief was confirmed by that doctor's response.

So, maybe I 'didn't do great', but being told that wasn't great, either.

According to the New Zealand College of Midwives, 'Traumatic birth experiences can have an impact on the initiation and establishment of breastfeeding, bonding and attachment between the mother and her baby, recovery from birth, and short- and long-term health challenges.'[10]

In August 2024, Catie McDonald told the *NZ Herald* that during the birth of her second child 'a midwife discovered the umbilical cord was compressed and prolapsing, so she was rushed in for an emergency C-section and put under general.[11]

"I had to say goodbye to my partner, they put a mask over my face and I went to sleep. I woke up a mother but I was so confused and upset… and totally out of it. I cried and cried and was told by the doctors that I should be so happy that I had a healthy baby. I really tried my best to be, but it took months."

And it took years to recover emotionally from the birth. Catie said that she is still upset when she thinks about it.

"I feel like that trauma ran alongside me, parallel to everything else in my life and was heightened in the quiet alone moments, which are fleeting as a young mother. Birth trauma stays with you for a long time, it has taken me years to be able to talk to people about Eve's birth without feeling really upset. Even now ... I get tears in my eyes thinking about her birth and the weeks that followed, because I know that the trauma affected my ability to bond and enjoy that newborn time with her."'

New Zealand College of Midwives midwifery adviser Claire MacDonald says 'community-based midwives were experts at primary care – including "holistic assessments of māmā and pēpi wellbeing throughout the postnatal period" – and could recognise when additional support was needed and offer referrals, but sometimes there were no support services available locally, or there were long waitlists.

"'A gap in service availability for mild to moderate mental health has been identified across the whole health service, including maternity."'[12]

CEO and founder of Birth Trauma Aotearoa, Kate Hicks, is quick to note that stigma and shame around birth trauma leads to it being under-reported and under-claimed for, further leading to fewer available trauma-informed supports in terms of psychological trauma.

'If a mum is experiencing significant distress, then the Maternal Mental Health service can support them ... Mum may be able to access support via her GP but many parents don't know these services exist.'

I don't know about you, but I only learned that there are trauma-informed support avenues available – for said psychologically machine-gun obliterated new mamas – when I read Kate's article. So I feel the damage is well and truly, irreversibly done and dusted now. I am mere ashes to ashes at this point.

Hicks does say that she would like to see 'a nationwide policy of at least one physical checkup and one psychological checkup available to every birthing parent following every birth, or loss, as standard practice in Aotearoa, including access to further care if needed.' If needed! Studies have shown that psychological trauma from birth causes new mums the same body and brain response as those who experienced natural disasters, war, or assault.[13] If I had to pick which category resonates most with my miraculous life-creating and excreting experience, it would be natural disaster, more specifically Naomi Watts in *The Impossible* – when the tsunami hits and she's rinsed, spun, rick-rolled and rag-dolled into another dimension, eventually bobbing back to the surface like a decimated little piñata, with a tree branch impaling her leg.

Thankfully, cover and counselling is now available for birth injuries – and of course it covers mental injuries due to birth trauma, too. And that's a huge win for the one-third of mothers that, statistics show, considered their birth psychologically traumatic – which equates to 50 mothers per day in New Zealand.[14]

Oh, but guess what: you are covered only as long as the diagnosis of a mental injury is deemed to be a consequence of a physical injury.

The following is the specified list of maternal birth injuries, occurring from the onset of labour to the postpartum period, that are now defined as personal injuries:

- Obstetric anal sphincter injury tears or tears to the perineum, labia, vagina, vulva, clitoris, cervix, rectum, anus or urethra
- Ruptured uterus during labour
- Obstetric fistula (including vesicovaginal, colovaginal and ureterovaginal)
- Anterior wall prolapse, posterior wall prolapse or uterine prolapse
- Coccyx fracture or dislocation
- Pubic ramus fracture
- Obstetric haematoma of pelvis
- Postpartum uterine inversion
- Levator ani avulsion
- Symphysis pubis capsule or ligament tear
- Pudendal neuropathy

The following maternal birth injuries, occurring from the onset of labour to the postpartum period, are NOT defined as personal injuries:

- No medical records state that on the operating table the mother couldn't breathe and was uncontrollably shaking so much her muscles had started to seize.
- The mother was given drugs that made her panic more.
- No medical records state that when this first-time mum woke up, she didn't ask to hold her baby because she didn't actually even remember there was a baby and was instead convinced she had already failed motherhood – just minutes into it.
- Medical records do state the operation had gone smoothly; the baby was perfectly okay and healthy.
- The mother was later told by a medical professional, present at the birth, 'Yeah look, I'll be honest. You did okay. But you didn't do great.'

1 AUGUST 2023, 10:43 P.M.

Sinead: [Image]

Sinead: Hehe!!!!!

Sinead: Meet Vivieeeee

Sinead: She can't wait to meet her aunty Amyyyy xxx

Sinead: Are my messages coming through??

Sinead: Thought u wuld really want to know shee's arrriiived! Xoxox

Amy has seen this message.

I don't want to go to Birthcare, I want to go to the clubs

THE NIGHT I HAD VIVIE I ASKED STU TO ORDER AN UBER so we could go clubbing in Ponsonby, and he had to remind me I was paralysed from the waist down. I told him that was fine and to just fetch me a wheelchair and a chilli margarita from the cafeteria – which obviously they don't serve – and I'd be ready to rock and roll.

I felt high as a fucking kite, like I had taken ecstasy. I don't know if it was the post-birth hormones, the morphine drip I was hooked up to or the fact I'd just held down a footlong chicken and bacon ranch sub – the first food I hadn't violently thrown up in nearly a year.

Like a normal person who had just had a baby and a normal person who had just been born, Stu and Vivie ignored me and fell asleep. So, I stayed awake near-gurning from 8 p.m., sending crazed messages to nearly every one of my hundreds of Facebook contacts announcing I had 'Just had a baby!! 😀'. The ones I was actually friends with congratulated me. Those who were an old high-school classmate or aunt's neighbour understandably left me on seen (I'd met my stepdad's friend's ex-girlfriend Amy once about 25 years earlier).

At around midnight, when all those poor people had gone to sleep, I started messaging all my contacts (nope, not 'friends' – simply anyone in my phone contacts) who lived in different time zones, informing them of the exciting news they didn't give one shit about.

At 8 a.m., both Stu and Vivie woke to me grinning at them, mania in my eyes. Stu said 'dear God,' and ordered me to go to sleep. I refused.

I was no longer sick.

I was free.

I was reborn.

I was carpe diem.

I was Livin' la Vida Loca.

And I never needed to sleep again, thank you.

When a nurse came in to remove my catheter, I said I don't know why people say C-sections suck, I felt perfectly fine and dandy. She reminded me I was hooked up to morphine, and that it was time to disconnect me. The party was over.

After we were discharged we moved to Birthcare, which is exactly when the morphine wore off – when I had my tiny brand-new baby in a moving car, with lots of other moving cars around that I knew would smash into us and she would definitely die. So, while we drove over every speedbump and I screamed as my stitches were jostled, I gripped her leg, just waiting for our car to get totalled. Fun!

Much to my surprise we made it to Birthcare with my stitches intact, and, even more surprisingly, a still-alive baby.

I had convinced Stu it was worth splurging on a premium room with a double bed that reclined, and it did feel like we were in an expensive hotel. Luxe linen, an ensuite, flat-screen TV and room service on tap. No dinner for me though, thank you Madame, just a bottle of your finest Syrah please.

The next few days were a blur of revolving midwives barging in to teach me how to breastfeed – each one giving contradictory advice and different techniques to the one before – and family and friends popping in to meet the baby – visitors who I wanted to leave as soon as they stepped through the door. I begged Stu with my eyes to kick them out, but he didn't take the hint.

Learning how to breastfeed is painful and humiliating enough, but in front of visitors – in front of my in-laws! – it was excruciating. I didn't want them to look at me, I didn't want them to be there, I hated them all, especially the one who gripped my baby tight and jiggled her around far more aggressively than I felt comfortable with. I wanted to Beyblade spin-kick them out the door so no one could come in and touch my breasts or my baby ever again.

What should have been the best visit, from my best friend Hannah, was one of the worst. My obstetrician later said he had forgotten to warn me of shoulder tip pain (STP) from post-surgery trapped gas, as it's 'so rare, there's no way it would happen to you on top of HG!'.

As Hannah walked in the door, grinning ear-to-ear at meeting her god-daughter and new-mum best friend, I crumpled onto the bed gasping in agony. I know STP sounds, like, whatever, but people have compared it to the exact pain of a crocodile chomping its teeth down into your flesh. (If you haven't learned by now, I get every rare bad thing going – especially when it comes to having a baby. Thank God I have a sense of humour, because, honestly, how else would we cope?)

If I could go back and change one thing about those first few weeks – along with recognising earlier that my mental health was going down the drain – I'd put an absolute ban on visitors and just keep it to the three of us and her big brothers.

Later that day after the nap from hell, there must have been a shift changeover with the nurses and perhaps a dropped paper-trail with my meds. Specifically, laxatives. I appeared to have been double-dosed. In the middle of the night, I woke up knowing something very bad was about to happen. I heaved my sore, swollen body out of bed, whimpering in agony at my straining stitches, and dragged myself to the bathroom.

I forgot I couldn't lower myself onto the toilet without Stu's help (a true low point in our romantic relationship; he'd also been changing my blood-soaked nappies) and couldn't sit down. So, I shat all over the Premium Suite tiles.

In hindsight, of course, I don't know why I didn't push the call button for a nurse or wake Stu to help me. I think I thought he'd been through enough for the last nine months.

As hot tears poured down my cheeks from the pain, I attempted to wipe the shit off the tiles, change my clothes and crawl back into bed in shame.

Why is every part of childbirth horrific? Why can I never catch a break and not evacuate my bowels on the fancy floor after spending my entire pregnancy vomiting on every surface?

The day after I soiled the Birthcare floor, we went home. I made Stu take a photo of me holding tiny Vivie outside the Birthcare doors – a landmark pic every millennial new mum insists on. In it I'm wearing milk-stained pajamas in broad daylight. I posted it on Instagram to my five thousand followers – most of whom are strangers – with the caption:

'Ran out of clothes 'cause I shat myself, the miracle of life, mwah xx'

That was the first time I decided to start telling the truth on the internet, to help other mums who might have shit on tiles that cost $735 a night feel less terrible.

13 AUGUST 2023, 2:42 P.M.

Sinead: Hey guys hope you and babas all doing good – we must hang soon it's been literally years. Hey just messaging out of blue sorry as not doing great right now haha. Um just wondering if any of you guys started breastfeeding and then stopped because it hurt heaps? I'm struggling a bit and I'm so tired and I'm not sure when I last ate but maybe I should just push through, right?

Incoming group chat call from Dani. Sash and Anna have joined the call.

Sinead: Guys thank you so much for talking me through that. I've been in such a dark place and you all lifted me out. I'm so grateful. I'm so lucky to be in the mum club now and just be able to message any old random mum and she will help HAHA. And you are the best of the randoms. When I emerge from this newborn hell am taking you all out for chilli margs chahoo.

Sinead: [Image]

Sinead: Vivie says thank you for helping her mum stop crying <3

Dani: We love you. This shit is so hard. You're the best mama and I know Michele would be so proud of you. She always was. And I can't wait to meet Vivie and cuddle her and cuddle you. Xx

Sinead: Me too, as soon as my tits aren't fucking agony.

Anna: Please try to remember this is the hardest job in the world – but you're exactly the mama Vivie needs. You have always been so strong, and I know how strong you're being for her. We love you x

Sash: We're always here for you, we've all been through it, you're not alone. And despite how you feel, you're doing the most amazing job. Always always reach out when you feel like you're not and we will remind you.

Sinead: Thank you. I think I'll give it a couple more days and if it's still shithouse I'll stop breastfeeding, definitely.

14 AUGUST 2023, 11:14 A.M.

[Incoming call – Stuart Dye]

Han: Hey Stu! How's our gal pals today?

Stu: Han, it's not. It's not good over here. I don't, I don't...

[Ride confirmed. Anderson is arriving soon. 3M53AF. Silver Honda Civic]

Han: What's happening?

Stu: She. She won't get out of bed. I bring her food and she won't eat it. I bring Vivie to her and say, 'Look who wants to cuddle their mum!' and she won't take her. She won't look at her. She won't look at me. She just stares. At nothing. She's not looking out the window, she's staring out past it. I don't know what she's looking at. I don't... I don't know what to do.

Han: I'm eleven minutes away. Wait, about sixteen minutes – I just have to make a quick stop. Sixteen minutes. You tell her Han's coming, she just has to do sixteen minutes more, that's all.

If Breast Is Best then why do I hate her?

ON THE TWELFTH DAY AFTER HAVING VIVIE, I couldn't get out of bed anymore. I couldn't stop crying. Arms full of baby, Stu gently pleaded with me to come downstairs to be with them. But I couldn't move.

Breasts boiling hot and engorged, it felt like there were concrete slabs pinning me down. A breast pump sat on my bedside table, taunting me. I had tried and failed to use it – it hurt too much and the repetitive, heaving mechanical sound of it made me more anxious.

Thirty minutes later, my best friend Hannah walked into my dark, sweat-smelling bedroom with two bottles of wine in tow and climbed into bed with me. Handing me an RSA-worthy pour, she put her hands gently on mine and said 'We're stopping now. This ends now.'

I had spent nearly two weeks in pain, unable to hold Vivie on my chest or cuddle with Stu because my boobs hurt so badly. My hair was lank, itchy and greasy because I couldn't lift my arms over my head to wash it.

But my midwife had convinced me that breastfeeding was good for mums with mental illnesses, because it released oxytocin. I know now that while, yes, that might be true – particularly as I was in the throes of postnatal depression (PND) – being able to wash my hair, hold my child and partner, and have a wine would have been more beneficial for my mental health.

Formula had always been my backup plan – I wasn't opposed to it at all. When I was pregnant I had decided that I'd give breastfeeding a go, but that if I didn't like it, if it didn't come easily for us or if it started impacting my mental wellbeing, I'd stop immediately. But I hadn't known about the Birthcare posters.

Rather than a single brochure about the signs of PND to look out for, the ward was instead plastered with huge signs pushing 'Breast Is Best'. They outlined the tiny handful of ingredients that are apparently in formula alongside a mammoth list of the benefits of breastmilk – none of which were a mum who was in pain and hating her child.

I'd had a C-section, so my body was swollen with fluid, and consequently my milk was trapped. In the beginning I had pushed through it, even though Vivie latching on felt like a snake biting down on my nipple. What was supposed to be a bonding experience saw her hungry, frustrated and wailing – and me anxious, whimpering in pain, gritting my teeth while hot tears dripped onto the top of her head. But Breast Is Best right?

What was touted as a 'natural' way for us to connect meant I couldn't cuddle my baby or burp her – Stu had to do it every time. I was just too sore. And I felt left out, useless and detached from both of them.

What these posters claimed was an easy, convenient way to feed my child meant that, instead of a simple bottle of formula, I had been carting a breast pump, nipple shields, ice packs, breast pads and nursing cups around the house – always forgetting something and having to heave my aching body back up the stairs to find it. It meant panicking that I was over-feeding or under-pumping and never getting it right.

Through all of it, I didn't understand how the supposed oxytocin release was making me the sickest I'd ever been.

Everyone told me to stop: Stu, my mum friends, even friends from high school who I hadn't seen for ages but have since had babies. I don't know why I didn't listen. Maybe I needed Hannah to give me permission to stop. Maybe I needed someone who wasn't a parent but who loves me as much as a parent does, who cared more about me than this brand-new baby, to tell me fuck the oxytocin, fuck the alleged benefits of breastfeeding – and to tell me that Vivie needed a healthy mum more than she needed breastmilk.

My whirlwind relationship with breastfeeding was over.

Now exclusively formula-fed, Vivie has about seven chins, and Plunket has suggested she is 'over-fed.' She's the fattest baby in my antenatal group and has worn size two clothes since she was six months old. She's so fat. She's perfect.

When chef and dad of five Jamie Oliver commented that women should breastfeed because 'it's easy, it's more convenient, it's more nutritious, it's better, it's free,' singer Adele, a new mum at the time, wasn't having a bar of it.

'It's fucking ridiculous, and all those people who put pressure on us, you can go fuck yourselves, alright?' she retorted publicly during a concert in London.

'Because it's hard. Some of us can't do it. I managed about nine weeks with my boobs ... Some of my mates got postnatal depression from the way those midwives were talking. Idiots.'

'Breastfeed if you can but don't worry, [formula milk is] just as good ... All I wanted to do was breastfeed and then I couldn't and then I felt like, "if I was in the jungle now back in the day, my kid would be dead because my milk's gone."'[15]

And after the birth of her second child, Banks, Hilary Duff shared her gripe with Breast Is Best messaging on social media.[16]

'I am a working mom of two ... Pumping at work sucks ... Even if I had the luxury to be in my own room, it's not even considered a 'break' because you have to sit upright for the milk to flow into the bottles! Plus, you are having your damn nipples tugged at by an aggressive machine that makes an annoying sound, that echoes through your head day and night ...'

'Ttttthen having to find some place to sterilize bottles and keep your milk cold ... I needed a break. I was going to break. With the stress of a dropping milk supply and a baby that was getting bored or not caring about nursing when I was available to. I was sad and frustrated and feeling like a failure all the time.'

Shortly after I threw in the towel on breastfeeding, I shared a post on Instagram outlining my struggles with it and my hatred of those Birthcare posters. The post went viral, reaching nearly 10,000 people – two of which were my midwife and obstetrician. My midwife would go on to apologise for making me feel pressured to breastfeed, but I assured her that it wasn't her – it was the Breast Is Best messaging everywhere new mums look.

After quitting breastfeeding, both Hilary Duff and actress and comedian Amy Schumer shared their experiences.

'I am happy to say that I haven't fed or pumped in three days and it's crazy how fast you can come out on the other side,' wrote Duff.

'[I feel] fine and happy and relieved and silly that I even stressed on it so hard. Banks is thriving and I get even more time with her and daddy gets to do more feeds! And mommy gets a tiny bit more sleep.'[17]

Schumer said she tried pumping for a month after her son Gene wouldn't latch and then called it a day.

'Some people just absolutely love it and I'm so happy for them. But it was just bumming me out ... once it occurred to me that I could stop. I was like, "I'm going to stop." ... You matter, and it's going to be better for your baby that you're okay.'[18]

A week after I quit, one of my Instagram followers told me Birthcare had taken the signs down. I never found out whether that was because of what I shared – which led to many people making complaints – or if it was just a coincidence.

I like to think my post made a difference, even a tiny one. Maybe not with the signs, but with just one hurting, miserable mum somewhere in New Zealand, hunched over, trying to feed a hungry and miserable baby. I like to think maybe her partner called in their version of Hannah, who took her hands, fed her sips of wine and told her that she's been through enough now.

17 AUGUST 2023, 3:14 P.M.

Sinead: I have arrived at my padded cell

Hannah: That actually sounds very cosy? How are you feeling though, for real?

Sinead: I feel sad. For Stu and for Vivie, that I'm a fuck-up wife and an even worse mum

Hannah: You are not a fuck-up, you just need some help to get through this and that's what you're doing. It's an incredibly selfless thing to do, and very responsible to recognise that this is the right choice for you to get healthy.

Sinead: K but may we discuss they only let in the three most mentally fucked mums in the northern regions here??

Hannah: You are excelling!! For the first time in your life you are top of the class.

Sinead: They took my phone charger! Like, it's 50cm long and I'm five foot – do they think I'm gonna get all the other inmates to human pyramid me up close enough to the ceiling that I can hang myself with this tiny string?

Hannah: I love you so much. You are doing all the best things to be the best ma and wife. And thank god phones don't have cords on them anymore, so your burner is safe.

Hannah: youtube.com > Akon > Locked Up. Thinking of you x

Hannah: Also, this is your very own Girl, Interrupted moment? You could write a book on this one day and make your millies.

A week in the clink: what it's like to be hospitalised with PND

'WELL, IF YOU WEREN'T DEPRESSED BEFORE you sure as shit will be now,' my husband laughed. But the laughter was hollow.

Earlier that day my midwife had told me she thought I'd be sent to a lovely respite centre out in West Auckland. She had shown me pictures of the accommodation – cute little brick cottages with cosy rooms fitted out with cream linen armchairs, white wooden cots and ensuite bathrooms.

I was nervous about going somewhere I'd never been before, on my own with our two-week-old baby, but thought the centre looked nice – like it would be restorative. I assumed it would be like that wellness retreat Nicole Kidman ran in *Nine Perfect Strangers*, and me and other mums would don robes and drink green tea and do healing circles.

But that was not where I was sent when postnatal depression stuck its claws deep inside me.

Much like her birth, I don't remember much from the first week after Vivie was born. I remember being delighted that I could hold food down for the first time in nearly a year, but the rest is a blur of attempting to breastfeed and hating it, countless visitors at Birthcare that I wanted to leave as soon as they arrived, and a baby in a bassinet next to me that was a total stranger.

She didn't look how I imagined she would. Now as I write this, with my laptop on one knee and her sleeping in my lap, she's the chubbiest three-month-old in my mums' group – with cheeks so big she looks like a chipmunk. She's identical to how I looked at her age, and exactly what I thought she'd look like.

But she was slim and dainty when she was born, with an elfish face I didn't recognise – probably because she was born early. I had pleaded for a C-section at thirty-eight weeks because I couldn't go on any longer; I had been in hospital on an IV drip for dehydration every few days and was mentally exhausted.

While I felt a duty to care for her, I also felt like I was babysitting and that her real mum was coming to pick her up at some stage. Even now, three months on, I still often feel like I'm playing house. When I take her for walks in her pram, I'm convinced people think I'm the nanny.

A week after we got home from Birthcare, I started getting sick again. My initial post-birth oxytocin high had worn off – I had constant headaches, I was either freezing cold or drenched in sweat, and my vomiting came back.

I became convinced that there must have been a complication with my C-section, that perhaps they had left an instrument inside that was poisoning me.

When my daughter woke me crying in the night, I simply could not get up to feed her. I was confined to bed, paralysed by the sound. I would put earplugs in and pretend I couldn't hear her.

My husband took over looking after our daughter in the night so that I could sleep and try to get better. But despite sleeping twelve hours a night – unheard of for a mother with a newborn – I would wake up more exhausted than the day before.

I remember crying to my husband saying something was wrong with me – but as a third-time dad, a literal old hand, he tried to reassure me that 'this is just what having a newborn is like, you're supposed to be tired'.

It wasn't until his mother came to meet the baby that my pleas were taken more seriously: she told him he needed to take me to the doctor because my skin was grey and I 'wasn't right'.

One of my mum friends also stepped in and confirmed this wasn't normal. She explained that mothers are biologically programmed to be able to get up to feed their babies in the night – no matter how tired they are – and that the fact I couldn't meant something was wrong.

My husband took me to a GP, who checked me over thoroughly and said nothing was physically wrong with me. That's when I burst into tears, convinced she was missing something, convinced I was being poisoned and I was going to die. She hugged me and told me I needed to go see my psychiatrist – that this was likely a mental-health issue. I cried harder, saying she was wrong, because I wasn't sad, I was sick.

'What about the headaches? And the vomiting?' I cried.

We went straight to my psychiatrist. It took less than five minutes for her to diagnose me as suffering postnatal depression. It was severe, she said, and she was calling Starship Hospital to arrange a bed for me in the Mother and Baby Unit (MBU). Not the lovely brick cottages with linen rocking chairs for mums who just need a bit of R & R; a specialist unit, with only three beds for the mums with the most critical cases of PND in the northern regions. A unit where babies are admitted as patients as well, tiny victims of a condition that affects about 15 per cent of new mums.

On arriving at the ward, I had to hand my bags over for inspection, like at airport security. They combed through my possessions, including my daughter's tiny onesies. They took away sharp objects (RIP my nail scissors) and all medications and even confiscated my phone charging cord. They reluctantly gave it back to me a few hours later after I assured them I wasn't suicidal, in fact I wasn't even depressed – I was just sick, remember?

My husband and I were then given a tour of the facility. While I understand the public health system is horrendously underfunded and they had obviously done as much as they could to make the ward cosy, it was worlds away from the respite centre my midwife had shown me, let alone the townhouse Stu and I had lovingly furnished when we moved in two years ago.

The 'living room' was similar to a hostel's – a shared kitchen and bathroom, a couple of worn-out couches, a TV and a few toys for the children that had to stay there with their mothers. The 'outdoor area' was a patch of grass overlooking a construction site and a carpark.

My room was small: two single beds with just a hospital sheet on each, a single window, a changing table and a bassinet. It felt like a prison cell. And I felt guilty for thinking that when I knew I was lucky to be in a ward that could only take in three mums at a time.

On a different floor of the hospital, where I had delivered my daughter two weeks earlier, the heating had been cranked up high to keep the babies warm – so I had expected the same here and had arrived in a t-shirt and shorts. But the heater in my room was apparently broken and it was freezing. I would later spend the night walking out to the nurses' station every hour to ask for blankets, only to be given more sheets. I understand that's probably because they're easier to launder between patients, but that knowledge didn't help the fact my husband and I shivered all night – despite pushing the beds together and gripping onto each other, pretending we were back home in our California King.

Dinner had been a piece of fish and mashed potatoes, which was cold by the time we were brave enough to venture out into the living room. I didn't eat. I made jokes instead.

At this stage we were both still laughing at how dire it all was, because if you don't laugh, you'll cry, etc., and it truly was so grim it was almost funny.

For a while.

In hindsight, I think I was the one that kept cracking the jokes because I was trying to make the whole experience feel like an inane sitcom episode. Despite how awful it all was, I was trying with all my might to make it as fun as humanly possible for my husband, because I felt so guilty. Guilty I had made him spend a fortune on IVF. Guilty I had not been able to contribute financially to our family for a year because I'd been so sick. Guilty that instead of cuddling on the couch with our newborn baby, he was now in a depressing psych ward with a wife who couldn't get her shit together, who was always costing him money and causing him problems.

The next morning, I met the psychiatrist. She was going to start me back on the medications I was on before I fell pregnant, before I was pulled off them because they weren't pregnancy safe. I swallowed my pills then insisted I was fine to go home now, 'I promise'.

She explained that while I was free to come and go as I pleased, they highly recommended I stay a few days 'just to talk a bit and get some rest'. I ignored their recommendation.

I didn't belong there anyway! I was fine – definitely fine now I had my meds back.

The staff were reluctant to discharge me but let me leave under the condition that my husband did not leave me home alone at any time.

We went home that afternoon, but the next day, in an attempt to ease some of my guilt, I convinced my husband he should go to the pub to catch up with friends and blow off some steam and that 'I was fine'. Just an hour after he left, my two-week-old fell off the couch while I was in the kitchen making bottles. I called an ambulance and we were rushed back to Starship – but this time to the ER.

As a doctor examined our daughter, asking us questions on how the accident happened, I turned away and left my husband to answer while I scrolled Instagram. Stu was understandably disturbed by this behaviour, but I explained through tears it was because I was so terrified they thought it wasn't an accident that I was scared of saying the wrong thing.

'Well, scrolling through Instagram while they question you isn't a great look, then,' he said.

He seemed angry but I know now he was scared. He, too, had thought that when the baby was finally born, I wouldn't be sick anymore and he would have his wife back.

My phone rang. It was one of the nurses from the MBU, checking in to see how my day was going. I explained what had happened – that I had only turned my back for a second and Vivie fell – while sobbing and begging her not to take my baby away.

The nurse reassured me that one accident absolutely didn't mean I was in trouble, and that no one was taking my daughter anywhere.

They asked to speak to Stu and told him that while they couldn't force me, they strongly recommended I be readmitted to the ward for a few days, particularly after such a distressing accident. They were worried about what it would do to my already out-of-control anxiety and feelings of failure as a mother. They also explained that if I returned to the ward, they would be able to accelerate my meds to a higher dose much faster than if I was at home – where they couldn't monitor me.

After six hours of observation, our daughter was given the all-clear – she was okay and thankfully hadn't suffered any injuries from the fall. We went home and I packed my bags for my second stint in the MBU.

This time, I came prepared: duvet, dressing gown, slippers, essential oil diffuser, eye mask and laptop. All the home comforts. But my husband couldn't stay with me this time – he had to be home with our other children. When it came time for him to leave the ward to pick the boys up from school, he hugged me tight and cried.

I was silent. I felt abandoned and resentful.

The next few days and nights blurred into one. I locked myself in my room with our baby, watching Netflix on the laptop, only creeping out to the kitchen when I needed to make up formula. I was smiley and charming to the nurses, convinced that with my beguiling smile and 'utterly sane' small talk in my Peter Alexander silk pajamas and designer slippers they would soon realise I didn't belong there.

The nurses agreed to look after my daughter during the night so I could catch up on sleep. That had been one of my non-negotiable terms on returning to the ward. I remember waking up with a headache around 3 a.m. during one of those nights and going out to the nurses' station to ask for Panadol. I saw a man I'd never met before sitting on one of the couches, feeding my baby a bottle. I walked back to my room. One of my mum friends later said she couldn't comprehend how I could leave my baby with a stranger and just walk away, and I replied, 'because at the time I thought she was probably better off with him than me.'

Another night, one of the nurses helped me give my daughter her first bath. While she gently led the routine, she asked me to check the temperature of the water. When I said I didn't know, but I thought it felt okay, she grinned at me and said 'See, you do know. You know your baby, and you're doing a great job.' I felt five years old with my first report card, a big sticker and an A+.

On one of the days, my friend Anna came to visit us in the ward. She had flown over from Sydney and we had been planning her visit for months. We were meant to spend the afternoon on my deck, drinking rosé and eating a cheese platter.

I called her the day before she was due to arrive and explained where I was, that plans had changed, that I was so sorry. When she arrived at the ward, she looked sad and nervous, like she was visiting someone very sick in hospital.

Then I remembered that she was.

I felt ashamed that I had brought her here. I pride myself on being a great host, and this wasn't what we had planned. But 'come in anyway, sorry about the mess'. I took her to my little room, and she gave me a box of presents for me and my daughter: new fluffy slippers, chocolates, relaxation tea, face masks and a little baby book and rattle – plus a stack of frozen dinners her Auckland-based mum had made for my family.

While I perched on the edge of the bed, she sat in a rocking chair near the window, holding my daughter. Whenever people come to visit new babies, they want a photo to share, so I took one of them together and sent it to her.

'That chair kind of looks like the one we have in the lounge at home so it's fine for you to post; no one will know where I actually am,' I said.

'No, it's not for Instagram,' she said. 'It's just for me, so I can look at it all the time and think of her and think of you.'

That's when I stopped trying to be a great host.

Instead, I lay down on the bed and quietly watched my great friend cuddle my baby with the sun shining down on their faces.

On the last day of my stay in the MBU, the psychiatrist said that my medication dosage was now at a high enough level that I could go home. I called Stu excitedly, and he said he'd pick me up as soon as he could leave work.

I packed my bags, put my daughter in her car seat and sat on the edge of the bed waiting to be collected.

Then the nurse who had phoned to check in with me on the day we were in the ER came to my room and told me the plan had changed, and that I had to tell my husband that I needed to hang around for a few more hours because there was 'some discharge paperwork to organise.' I'd soon discover that she was trying to stall our departure.

She wanted a chance to talk to me alone – without my husband around and me desperately trying to make the whole nightmare silly and fun.

'Sinead, you're so charming, and you're so funny – you're an absolute pleasure to have here. But I can see that behind that lovely smile and the jokes, you're a very sick girl – and I need you to be real with me now.'

That's when I cracked.

I'm not good at lots of things, but I am a really good communicator – it's my whole job. I'm not shy, I'm confident and I tell the truth, and I ask for help when I need it. I had told the truth this entire time; I had told all those people over and over again that I actually didn't feel very well at all. And when help came, I told those helpers the truth – that the help wasn't helping and that I was actually feeling quite a lot worse.

But they always said, 'you're doing really, really well.'

It's hard to remember exactly when, but maybe one of those days I remembered that I'm also so charming and so funny and maybe that will make them like me, so they'll really want to help me. Somehow, I still ended up there and I didn't know why. But I think she was the why.

She held my hand while I cried. I told her that maybe I didn't love my baby, and maybe I never would, because she'd made me so sick. I told her that whenever I carried Vivie down the stairs, I gripped the handrail with all my strength because I was so worried about slipping and dropping her – but that I also sometimes had intrusive thoughts of hurting her, and that I felt like a monster.

I told her that while I initially thought having a baby with someone who already had kids would be great because they'd know what to do, in reality it meant every time Stu gently critiqued how I was changing nappies or swaddling our baby – trying to be helpful of course – it landed like a brick and shattered what was left of my already dwindling confidence as a mother.

When my husband arrived, the nurse took him away for a 'quick chat'. I think she must have told him that right now, I needed lots of praise to build my confidence up. Critiques weren't life or death; they could wait till I was in a better place and better equipped to receive them.

We went home.

A few months later, my intrusive thoughts were more manageable. I was taking my meds every day. And my daughter had started laughing and smiling and only wanting to be held by me – and I think that's when I really started to love her. I think I needed her to show me she loved me before I could let myself love her.

One day, I want to raise money for the MBU to help more mums like me. I want to buy them nicer couches and duvets for the rooms. I want to take my baby back to see that amazing nurse, to show her how big Vivie's gotten – and show her I'm better now. Most of all, I want to thank her for seeing me.

8 FEBRUARY 2020, 1:12 P.M.

Sinead: Can we discuss how I just went to work in a crop top, cat eye and gold hoops, even though I WASN'T EVEN ROSTERED ON – just in the hopes my work crush would ask me for a drink.

Kate: *all capslock* Sinead, get out of work. I'm sending you straight to Gloriavale. Also, who's the crush?

Sinead Corcoran has sent a picture.

Kate: Who is this man? We shall pick this up this tomorrow. As if we were a fortune 500 company about to sit for their monthly board meeting. Add it to the agenda.

How he met your mother

23 FEBRUARY 2020, 3:54 P.M.

Sinead: I'm trying to write these recaps of The Bachelorette and I don't want to put my name on them because I want this guy to think I am a proper serious journalist. Also, he's not like my boss-boss, he's only my boss on the weekends and I only work every fourth weekend and only on Saturdays and I can't do maths but that seems like not very much my boss so maybe it's fine to be his girlfriend? It has to be fine because I can't stop thirsting after him Kate. But also do I love him or can I just not be bothered going on real dates anymore, so I've just developed a crush on whoever or whatever I see around the office?

28 FEBRUARY 2020, 6:32 A.M.

Sinead: Good morning. I pashed my boss.

Kate: I'm screaming? Tell me everything obviously.

Sinead: *no punctuation, no time for that* We had our readership result drinks last night and then went to the pub and we were obviously the last two there and he was like look I promise I'm only going to ask this one time and if you say no I promise I'll never ask again and I'll quit and

I'll flee the country if you want but I was wondering if I could take you out to dinner sometime and I was like okay first things first are you my boss or no and he said no only technically if you happen to be working a Saturday which you only do one day a month so I'm only your boss like 2% of the time maybe I can't do maths.

Kate: That's hot.

Sinead: And then we talked for like three hours and I'm not sure what happened but now we're getting married and having a baby, I think? And then said 'would it be okay if I kissed you?' And I said 'yes'. But that first kiss was like, very dainty? Like a very small moth gently landing on my lips? Is this a British thing? Or because he's quite old maybe? Is this how old people kiss? Like moths?

Sinead: Anyway, I took things over from this moth man so then we properly pashed in the street and now I'm doing no work because I can't stop thinking about it.

9 MARCH 2020, 8:17 A.M.

Sinead: Okay I actually think we're in love, and it's been 11 days. Do we think it's fine I'm going to marry a 44-year-old?

Kate: Absolutely, you'll be like Calista Flockhart and Harrison Ford, Or Catherine Zeta-Jones and Michael Douglas.

ANZAC DAY, 25 APRIL 2020, 5:35 P.M. LOCKDOWN.

Sinead: Okay so me and Stu are both working at the dining room table and Stu is the home page editor tonight so is technically my boss. And he goes 'Hey this is awkward, but maybe can you do some work? Because I can see you're just online shopping?' Like lol Stu what are you going to do, fire me? OK good luck Weinstein.

My wonderful wife is cursed, by Stuart Dye

MY MUM AND DAD CAME TO VISIT US at home when Vivie was about 10 days old. They'd been to the hospital and to Birthcare for the first glimpses of their seventh grandchild, but this was the first time to see us all in our natural habitat; in the glow of newborn bliss, cuddled together on the couch, tired but smiling.

Mum grabbed Vivie for a snuggle and asked how I was doing as Sinead showered upstairs. There's a well-worn schtick for this kind of conversation in our family. I smile and say everything is terrific then freeze my face in mock horror. Mum and Dad laugh. I break the joke and say, 'yeah I'd forgotten how exhausting it is, but you know, you just get on with it and we're doing fine'.

Sinead comes downstairs and I know Mum and Dad will hug her and tell her she's doing great. They'll tell her she's shattered and that's to be expected but everything will get better bit by bit. Sleep when the baby sleeps, and all that.

Instead, they seem to freeze.

They push through the motions of a hug, cluck over Sinead and the baby, and sound the platitudes, but I can tell something isn't sitting right. I try to take stock through the fog of sleeplessness but can't put my finger on the source of the tension. Sinead battles to engage in conversation for half an hour then goes upstairs for a lie-down.

Mum: 'Stuart, something's not right.'

Me: 'We're fine. It just is what it is. Exhausting, but everyone goes through this phase, right?'

Mum: 'Sinead is grey. She can hardly speak. She needs help. Stuart, you need to get her help.'

Is it the British stiff upper lip? In New Zealand 'she'll be right' is the same crime by another name. Clichés are only clichés because they are true. Then again, is that an excuse I give myself for failing when I was needed most? The mirror of self-reflection isn't always clear.

What is clear now is that – to seize another cliché – I couldn't see the wood for the trees.

I default to looking on the bright side and finding the humour in any situation, no matter how black. In the case of Sinead's deteriorating mental health, it was a dangerous default.

Sinead had a series of symptoms which, taken individually, could be passed off with a laugh about how tough the newborn phase is.

Exhausted? Which new parents aren't?!

Struggling to bond? Not surprised – the baby doesn't do anything but feed and sleep!

Feeling down? That's why they call it baby blues!

No appetite? Who has time to eat anyway!

Anxiety? That's nothing new!

And on and on and on.

Taken collectively these were red flags that, in hindsight, couldn't have been more obvious if Sinead were holding a sign saying 'I have postnatal depression'. Yet even once I understood what it was, I felt powerless. What do I say to her? Who do I turn to? Is there medication? Does she need therapy? What do I say to people who ask me how we're doing? What does our future now look like?

I was helpless and I was hopeless.

It wasn't the first time I'd felt this way. When Sinead was 29 her 'brain broke', as she likes to put it. I was out watching football and she kept messaging saying she wasn't feeling good. I didn't hurry – it was England in the Euros final, which surely took precedence. By the time I got home she was in a bad way. She kept insisting things didn't feel real. I told her everything was real. She asked if I was real.

What followed was a whirlwind of A&E, misdiagnosis, doctors' appointments, an ill-fated attempt at a birthday weekend of R&R and a scuppered plan to propose to her. A crisis appointment with a psychiatrist and, ultimately, referral to community mental-health service the Taylor Centre. It was a steep learning curve to comprehend anxiety, dissociation and its myriad varieties, triggers and potential treatments.

It took months to get back on an even keel. Given that history just two years earlier, it seems bizarre now to think that I was so lost once again.

After Mum's intervention, we made a rapid-fire appointment with the doctor. Sinead had become convinced something physical was badly wrong. She was sleeping 12 hours a night and still napping for several hours each day. I was trying to be understanding – but I was also getting frustrated at doing every night with Vivie and then most of the day. I was tired too. I wanted to yell at her. I'm ashamed writing that now.

The doctor was gentle but made it very clear there was nothing physically wrong. She suggested a psychiatrist might be worth talking to so it was back to our old friends at the Taylor Centre. (As an aside, the people who work there are remarkable in the face of a woefully underfunded service and an onslaught of urgent need.)

We went straight from the doctor to Sinead's psychiatrist, who took one look at her and called the hospital to have her admitted to a specialist mum and baby ward.

We arrived at the ward that evening. 'God, if you weren't depressed before we got here you certainly will be now.' My attempts to avoid resorting to jokes are still a work in progress.

Making light of things is a somewhat trite coping mechanism but it works for me. It helps me remember life isn't to be taken too seriously and it stops me falling into despair. I think it also stops me becoming angry. There are times when postnatal depression made me raging angry. It felt so unfair for Sinead to have to go through it after such an awful pregnancy - and, yes, I felt it was unfair on me too. It's all but impossible to be angry with an invisible foe so of course there were times when that anger was directed at Sinead. Why can't you just snap out of it? Millions of mums are doing it around the world; why can't you? I may as well be telling a blind person to look a bit harder, or ordering someone with a broken arm to put in a bit more effort to lift a barbell. We still largely treat mental illness as imagined, rather than in the way we treat conditions affecting other parts of the body. The brain is an organ and things can go wrong with it just as they do with a kidney.

I stayed with Sinead and Vivie in hospital that night. We had to hand over our phone charging cords; it took me a beat to realise why. A woman in the room next to us kept screaming. It was cold and desperately, desperately sad.

It sometimes seems my wonderful wife is cursed.

She bounced back from her 'brain breaking' but it took a long time. And part of the recovery was understanding there is no cure - this is a condition, likely to be lifelong, which needs to be managed. We both got better at that, so when a dissociative spell appeared it was less panic and more 'hello darkness my old friend'. Sinead took a bit of time away from work as it was a proven trigger for anxiety. When we got engaged, we (well, she) planned our wedding, and we got married and then decided we were in a good place to try for a baby through IVF, and we got pregnant straight away.

Oh, welcome to the party, hyperemesis gravidarum.

The first time Sinead vomited it was so exciting. It confirmed what we hoped - there was a baby on the way. By the time she was vomiting 20 times a day it wasn't quite so exciting. There were times she would drag herself to the kitchen sink, spewing on the floor part way there, and I would keep watching TV as I had become so immune to the sound (sorry for this, but immune to the smell as well).

Writing that, I realise how appalling it is that I could stare at a TV show as my wife retched and gagged a few feet away. I shouldn't have allowed that complacency anywhere near our lives – I know for sure that Sinead never had the luxury of becoming immune to her body racking over the sink or toilet bowl.

It was a profoundly difficult nine months culminating in a shambles of a delivery.

It's a sharp and confronting learning curve when it sometimes feels like you've become a full-time carer instead of a lover. The best advice I got was to understand the difference between sympathy and empathy. Sympathy is standing at the top of the pit (or sitting in front of the TV?) and sending pity vibes and words of encouragement down to the poor wretch below us. Empathy is clambering down into the pit, holding that person tight (holding her hair and rubbing her back if needed) and listening.

When you google 'advice for caregivers/partners of person with mental illness' everything says it's crucial to regularly take breaks for yourself, escape for a couple of hours to do some self-care and lean on friends for support. And better still, vent to them to get everything off your chest.

This sounds great in theory ... but I'm British, a man and 49, and unlike my wife I have no culture of FaceTiming my friends three times a day to talk about God knows what. Going to therapy and taking sertraline, or whatever, are still largely alien concepts. I'd sooner scrape my nails down a chalkboard than say things like 'hold space for their sadness' or 'lean in to it'. I was conditioned to think 'Right, no point wallowing – let's get on with it'.

So, in the throes of that nine-month-long nightmare, I didn't talk to anyone beyond an 'oh you know, it's really tough' when people asked how Sinead was. And even now, a year on and knowing how helpful it would have been if I had leaned on friends, it's still rare that I will, despite my wife's encouragement to 'talk shit about her, get it out'. We're constantly trying to drill into the boys how critical it is to talk about their feelings and be in touch with their emotions, but I do wonder if I'll ever get there – and it worries me that that might impact the children.

Instead of talking as much as I should, I play football – running around a field a couple of times a week with other middle-aged men who are probably kicking their shit out too.

Sinead has suggested finding one friend who has been through something similar to whatever I'm going through – whether that's a job loss, a sick wife or a mid-life crisis – and maybe try to talk to them, rather than with a group of mates. And that it doesn't have to be 'holding space' – it can just be a mate saying 'that's so shit'. That it's not wallowing, and that it's good for me.

I'm not there yet. I'm not sure many men are. But I'm trying. For the boys, for Vivie and for Sinead.

We never had the glowing newborn phase. In fact, it was pretty horrendous. But maybe that's not too bad. Sinead's 'brain break', bleak pregnancy and postnatal depression have put us in a totally different place to where I thought we'd be – but she's here and Vivie's here and there are a whole lot of other people I never knew we'd need.

We use practical steps, and the network Sinead has built around us. We make a list of all the things that might help. Breathing, exercise, talking, icepacks, watching *Friends* (yes, really. Every single episode). Sinead has all these in her toolkit, of course, but when she's in a bad way, she can't breathe let alone find the meditation app on her phone. (I now know the toolkit inside out and I have it in a Notes app on my phone to refer to). We call her GP to discuss medication and any changes he can suggest. We talk to her therapist, who brainstorms new ideas to reduce the panic and reassures us that this is temporary. We talk to Tom at the Taylor Centre, who is a beacon of support and helps arrange appointments with a psychiatrist. Her friends call three times a day to check in and distract her with jokes about how she's a lunatic. Her mum friends come over with their babies and take her for a walk to the park in the sun. We have help and we have hope.

As Vivie grows, I will try to remember everything I learned during her first few months. I'll try not to repeat the mistakes I made.

I will listen, listen, listen.

I'll remember that no one says 'I have postnatal depression' because no one has those words. What they might say is 'I don't feel great'. We need to listen, and we need to hear what that might mean. She won't always 'be right'.

I'll remember that in Vivie's first few months, I made the mistake of taking over and showing Sinead what to do – what I thought was helpful was in fact a toxic eroding of her confidence. I now try to be curious about what is happening for her – you don't have fix it; you just have to be there to listen and support.

I'll remember I must validate feelings and experiences – a new mum with PND doesn't need to hear to 'look on the bright side' or that 'hey, it will pass'; she needs to know that it's okay to feel terrible and that parenting is bloody hard and that you are there to help and not to judge.

And if she pushes me away – and I can't emphasise this one enough – I need to stay right where I am. It doesn't mean she doesn't want me there; it's just a symptom of this hideous condition.

I will tell her that this condition is not about weakness or not loving her baby and she can't just snap out of it.

I'll tell myself that she is not rejecting me but she is suffering.

I will watch her that bit closer – friends, family and medical professionals see her now and then, but I have a ringside seat to every tiny change and every warning sign, and someone struggling won't always tell you. I'll switch my default to err on the side of caution.

And I'll her she's doing a great job. I'll tell her Vivie won't be taken away. I'll tell her I'm there to help, that I'm proud of her and that I know she'll get better.

12 OCTOBER, 2023. 11:20 A.M. THE REAL MUM CLUB

Charlotte: What baby monitor do you guys all have?

Sinead: In theory we have the Babysense7 + Secure870 but I could never work out how to attach it to the corner of the SnüzPod?

Sinead: The first night I just tucked it into the corner of the Snuz and it must have fallen over because when I went to check my half of the walkie-talkie, she was a black lifeless lump, so I was like oh she's dead OK.

Sinead: So threw the monitor in the garage cause it was just too much of an emotional rollercoaster you know, so now we don't use a baby monitor cause like yes it was $800 and has hi-def sound and 19 lullabies on rotation, but can it do CPR? Prob no, so like what's the point – if she's dead she's dead.

She hasn't died yet, but she will soon

ON THE THIRD DAY AFTER VIVIE'S BIRTH, in the afternoon, Stu and I had drifted off into an exhausted slumber.

When I came to in a dark room, I let out a blood-curdling scream, heaving the blankets off me and shaking Stu awake. I thought we'd somehow been asleep for days and the baby was dead in her cot. He tried to calm me down, telling me we'd been asleep 15 minutes. Vivie was obviously okay, swaddled in her bassinet and snoring softly, but I was too far gone; shaking and sobbing.

This would not be the first time I believed she had died.

The baby-in-bed nightmare pattern is this really fun thing where you frequently wake up convinced that your baby has somehow become tangled in your duvet and been smothered to death. You might scream and cry, and thrash at both the bed and your partner. When fully awake, you will confirm that your baby isn't, in fact, lost in the bed; it is in its own bed and perfectly okay – but you will not be able to calm down and/or sleep again.

'Hallucinatory baby-in-bed nightmares and other vivid dreams of the baby in peril appear to arise normally in response to the acute maternal responsibilities and sleep fragmentation that are endured by new mothers,' wrote Dr Tore Nielsen of the Sleep Research Centre in Canada.[19] Because everything in the bubble of hell and beyond is something to be endured by mothers, it seems. It is one long endurance test.

Even now, ten months on, I'm still constantly convinced she's dead. When she tipped her head underwater during her first bath at home and coughed up a mouthful; every morning when I tiptoe into her room to get her out of her crib; in her car seat while eating a cracker; on the floor playing with any toy small enough for her to choke on. But weirdly, whenever I think she's died – which is about thrice an hour every day – my instant reaction is often relief instead of terror. Because if she was dead, I wouldn't have to worry about her dying anymore, you see. If it happened, the never-ending anxiety would be over and maybe I wouldn't feel sick with worry all the time anymore.

I wonder if this is somehow linked to what a therapist once told me I was experiencing after my mum died: 'anticipatory grief'. In a nutshell, that's the distress you might feel before an impending loss, like the death of someone you love. My mum was diagnosed with breast cancer when I was sixteen, and around my twenty-first birthday we were told it was terminal. I spent the next year in a constant state of both dreading her death and wanting her to die so it would all be over. After she died, when I was 22, I couldn't shake the feeling that something terrible was about to happen, like I was watching a car crash in slow motion. It was that feeling of being in the dentist's waiting room, and I would shake with fear all day, every day. A few months later I was put on antidepressants for anxiety for the first time (but not the last).

My feeling of anticipatory grief went away with time and with meds until I had a baby, when it came back strong – and now I'm just waiting for her to die all the time. I don't know if this is because of my underlying anxiety disorder, or if this is just part of being a parent?

As I write this, it's nearly 10 p.m. Stu is downstairs watching A Man Alone.

Whenever Stu gets any spare time to himself, which is perhaps once every financial quarter due to our litter of children, he chooses to watch A Man Alone. Yes, this sounds like a category of porn, and it surely is – but in this instance it's the term we've coined for the only genre of film Stu wants to watch: A Man Alone Seeking Vengeance. You know the kind. Liam Neeson or Jason Statham or Keanu Reeves is there. His wife is dead or his kid is missing.

And why are they always Alone? Where are their pals?

Sometimes it's because years ago someone wronged the man in some way, or his daughter was kidnapped – so then he fell down inside a whiskey bottle for a very long time, until he was able to claw himself out, and when he emerged, it was with longer dirty hair and a beard. This hair growth is important; it is the Leading Actor in the film. It's to illustrate to the viewer that an undetermined length of time has passed and he is now in such a bad way he no longer has the strength to maintain basic personal hygiene.

Which brings us to Vengeance. To signal that the Vengeance section of the movie is en route, we will be shown a scene of him dry-shaving his beard in a dirty mirror.

The Man will now embark on his mission to Seek Vengeance – and this Venge will be either getting revenge against whoever wronged him and/or trying to find whichever child was kidnapped.

Unfortunately, I do not know if the child is ever located because I never watch these movies past the beard-shaving scene – and when I say watch, I kind of listen while catching up on my admin (which is rotting on Temu).

So, Stu's downstairs Alone with the Man, and, if I crane my ear towards the stairs, it sounds like the Man's tracked down his daughter, who is always played by Dakota Fanning. Which means

Stu will be pootling up to bed soon, which means it's time for me to send the text I have sent every evening since the day we got home from Birthcare.

'Please refresh my water bottle and check Bean is OK.'

Outside of this book we never actually call our daughter Vivie. And we certainly never call her Genevieve. Despite agreeing when I got pregnant that I could pick the baby's name – because Stu had already had two turns at choosing kids names – he vetoed every single one of my suggestions.

My third favourite – Holiday – was met with 'Sinead, as if you can pull off having a kid called that. Do you think you are a celebrity? God, don't answer that please.'

My second favourite – James – was slammed because Stu is a hundred years old and doesn't understand that it's cool to give girls boys' names now (and I was also planning on doing the 'we're not raising our child with birth sex pronouns – they will tell us what their gender is' thing. Which of course if she does, fabbo – boy, girl, anything in-between is cool, Bean.).

But my favourite of all the names was Vivienne, Vivie for short, which I thought was very cute, French and elegant. Stu, however, said it sounded like a bleached-haired chain-smoker who works behind the bar at the Rovers Return and spends her days asking 'What canna get ya luv?' in her gravelly voice.

We back-and-forthed for eight months, never agreeing, until one day he said he came across the name Genevieve when model Kate Upton named her daughter, but nicknamed her Vivie. So, I agreed because I planned on exclusively calling her Vivie and, behind Stu's back, telling everyone that it's short for Vivienne (and to this day I still do). This is also because my worst enemy who I loathe is called Jen, so I refuse for Gen to be my child's nickname.

But I needn't have worried about her nickname becoming Gen, because her nickname is not Gen and it's not even Vivie; it's Bean, which is actually short for Beanis the Weenis. And as with all children's nicknames, we have no idea where it came from.

Anyway, back to now.

Stu, as he does every night, checked B.Weenis on his way to bed. And after groaning when I made him pause tonight's Lonely Vengeful Man to read this chapter, he learned why I won't do the check. If I go in to check on Bean on my way to bed, she'll probably be dead, and I won't be able to fall asleep, obviously, because my baby is dead and I'll never sleep again – or I'll sleep forever because I'd have to end my life because my entire life is her and she's gone now.

Even if I was brave enough to pop my head in and do the nightly check and she was, as she always is, snuffling and snoring soundly – alive and well – that would mean that if for some reason she goes on to die in the night, which she definitely will soon, it would be all my fault because I was the one who checked and deemed her 'all good, just sleeping, not dead, as you were,' – so then she would have died on my watch.

Ergo, Stu needs to do the check because if she dies on his watch, I think one day, far away, I would be able to forgive him. Especially because he's my only family so, if I left him – which statistically I would, as 80 per cent of marriages end in divorce following the loss of a child – I'd not only not have Bean anymore, I'd have no one.

So, if Vivie died on his watch, I could forgive him. But if she died on mine, I never could.

That's why I don't do the final night-time check on my own baby. I've never been able to.

According to research, the love you feel for your baby when you see them sleeping is due to a combination of factors, including the hormone oxytocin and the ability of babies to sense and smell their mother's presence, which calms them.[20] But I've never been able to experience the last part of my day being a moment of overwhelming love for my child, because I'm not in the room for her to sense and smell so she feels calm. I'm not there to see the last time my baby is both as big as she's ever been and the smallest she ever will be, because when I see her in the morning, she'll be bigger, and she'll never be that little again.

And because I can't go into her room and get all of that oxytocin goodness, instead the last part of my day is a different moment. While Stu sleeps soundly next to me, having checked Vivie and given the 'all-clear, still breathing' and trusting that, I have a moment, which is much longer than a moment, that consumes me until my sleeping pills eventually kick in.

And it's thinking, incessantly, 'will tonight be the night she dies?'

And then thinking that maybe I'll be a bit relieved if she did because she was going to die one night anyway and there's nothing I can do to change that. And if she was dead, I wouldn't have to worry about her dying anymore, you see.

6 AUGUST 2023, 7:16 A.M.

Sinead: Hey gal!! How's it going now you've escaped Birthcare? This is so fucked right x

Beth: Haha yeah, it's so crazy bringing him home!! But now he's arrived earthside it's like he was meant to be here all along you know? 🌎 👶 God but mum's here with all these frozen lasagnas and stuff she meal prepped and it's so annoying like we can't fit them all in the fridge so thanks mum, huge help LOL. And now she's turning the kitchen upside down baking god knows what. But when she isn't vacuuming under me for the tenth time that day like a psycho, I'm just getting all the newborn snuggles in I can xx How are you guys going eeeeep? <3

Sinead: Oh yeah that sounds so annoying wtf. Gah, tbh I'm on struggle street man. You had a C-section too, right? This all just feels impossible while recovering ay, like how am I meant to look after a baby on no sleep when I can't even look after myself, I can't even stand up straight because it hurts so bad that I cry. We got home yesterday and I'm so fried I can't really think straight, and everything hurts and it's kinda weird she's here haha. And honestly it was like, kinda the worst day of my life.

Beth: Oh no, what do you mean though? What happened?

Sinead: Oh no, nothing like. Happened. It's all good, was probably just tired haha.

Beth: Awww it's such a beautiful day outside today☀️

Seen

Oh, OK so I'm raising Hell!

I TRULY THINK INSTAGRAMMING A PHOTO of you holding your tiny baby's feet and captioning it 'just soaking up this newborn baby bubble bliss' should be illegal.

It was all I ever read in the lead-up to Vivie's birth, so I was absolutely fizzing for my pregnancy to be over and to enter the bliss bubble. I pictured cosy contact naps on the couch, dressing my little doll up in Jamie Kay outfits, dreamy milky night-feeds and slow walks around the neighbourhood in the sun with her nestled in the front pack.

And maybe some people do have this first-week experience.

I, however, did not.

Hot engorged boobs that felt like they'd been sliced open. A stomach that had been.

Recovering from a C-section – or any birth, I imagine – on shreds of sleep while a baby screams day and night is an indescribable hell nothing can prepare you for – and those cursed Instagram captions sure as shit don't. It's physically and emotionally crippling, which is why I assume our brains make us forget the pain of birth and the pain of those first few months.

I remember one evening when I naively and hilariously contacted a sleep consultant because Vivie wouldn't sleep in her bassinet, only on our chests. I assume that because she needed a gig, the sleep consultant told us she could absolutely begin to implement a sleep-training routine for her. Vivie was eight days old at the time.

I know now from the sleep consultant we went on to hire when Vivie was five months old that newborn babies cannot and should not be sleep-trained. Newborn babies do not even know they have been born, so of course they only want to sleep atop your warm, womb-like chest. I know now that you must just suck up the fact that you will not be able to sleep for fear of them toppling off you.

In a BabyCentre article advising parents on what they need to know about life with a newborn, one of the pieces of advice is 'although it sounds cheesy, love is all you really need.'[21] This is utter obscenity. Love is not all you really need.

What you need is people to do a drive-by, but instead of machine-gun fire, they fling frozen Farro dinners out the car window to your doorstep – never knocking and saying 'Yoohoo I'm here to visit the baby <3'. (Pals of newborn parents: never, ever, visit during the bubble of hell. Especially unannounced.)

You will also likely need sleeping pills because 'sleep when the baby sleeps' is the most pointless advice. You will only find yourself falling asleep when the baby is awake and then startling with a jolt because you have fallen asleep holding the baby and maybe it has plummeted to the floorboards. Then when the baby is asleep, you will swipe through Instagram or TikTok to grasp at a thread of connection to the real outside world. Or send 52 identical photos of the baby to friends who generously say 'aww' as if this is new, interesting content. Or you'll attempt to shower your distressingly foreign body. Or stare at the baby wondering if it likes you and panicking because what if their eyebrows are just like not coming ever? And even when you do sleep, the true nightmare is you will never actually sleep. You will merely doze, poised for the always looming 'any minute now' moment when the baby wakes, and then they're awake so thereby you're awake.

In 1964, Randy Gardner stayed up for 264.4 hours (that's about 11 days and 25 minutes) to win a science fair competition. During the experiment, his mental state was tracked through a series of cognitive and sensory tests. After two days without sleeping, he began to have problems repeating simple tongue-twisters and he stopped being able to identify objects by touch.[22] His senses seemed to heighten, and he became sensitive to strong smells (at one point, he said, 'Don't make me smell that, I can't stand the smell').[23]

By the fifth day, he was paranoid and hallucinating, and he soon started having trouble forming short-term memories. On the eleventh day, when he was asked to subtract seven repeatedly, starting with 100, he stopped at 65. When asked why he had stopped, he replied that he had forgotten what he was doing. And in 1997, the Guinness World Records stated they would no longer accept entries of longest period without sleeping due to the inherent dangers associated with sleep deprivation.

You can imagine, then, what months on end of sleep deprivation could do to a person.

We have always been – touch wood – incredibly lucky with Vivie's sleeping. After the first six weeks or so, she was down to just two wake-ups a night, 2 a.m. and 4 a.m. There seems to be no rhyme or reason as to why some babies sleep more than others, but I remember the nurses in the MBU told me that, strangely enough, almost every mum admitted has an angel baby. It's as though the babies can tell their mum is having a rough time and they need to go easy on her. And once we sleep-trained Vivie with Hattie Moleta – who was my utter lifeline in those early days, and every day since – she's slept virtually every night.

And I know if you have a child who is not a great sleeper, you may understandably loathe me at learning this, even though you will feel bad loathing me, because you know I surely deserve this after hyperemesis. You will still loathe me because it's not fair, and I understand – I loathe me on your behalf – and will now stop talking about what an amazing sleeper Vivie is.

On Vivie's one-week birthday I shared a post about how I wasn't actually in a newborn bliss bubble; that I didn't know what it was, that instead I was in the throes of a trial by fire. I wrote that I was in both physical and mental agony, and that the only thing getting me through was the thoughtfulness and attentive care of my close friends, and the fact that on her seventh day here, Vivie smiled at me.

This post went a bit viral. Not to be vain and act like I am the Jesus of modern mothers – I just think my posts go viral because there are not many out there telling the truth. After a few of these posts on newborn hell bubble, breastfeeding and the stigma around elective C-sections, I became a small-time 'mumfluencer.' Not the proper kind where I got paid a lot to promote products, just the kind where I'd write stuff and get messages from other mums going through the same sort of thing, telling me I made them feel less alone.

I am not a God believer, or into anything spiritual whatsoever apart from Temu. I don't know what a chakra is (and actually for a long time I thought people were just misspelling Shakira of 'Hips Don't Lie' fame) and I don't own crystals (I have however mused several times this year on trying crystal meth and whether that would be hugely beneficial in getting this book done or not). And I am certainly not a star sign person who says stuff like 'That's why I'm an introverted extrovert, because I'm a Gemini with a rising sun on a resting whippet.' But I really do think I was put on this Earth for a reason: to do this.

Because if I didn't do this – use all the bad stuff that has happened to me (and likely will continue to happen lol) to help people, women, mums – then what was it all for?

Because if I don't do this – write, which is the only thing I've ever been able to do as easily as (and sometimes easier than) simply breathing in and out – it's like it was all just a quite-bad-a-lot-of-the-time life. Like it was all for nothing and I went through it all for no reason. And I need to hold onto the hope that it was for something, even something little. The very idea of what would happen – how I'd keep fighting – if that candle of light, of hope, flickered out frightens me.

On those burning-the-candle-at-both-ends days – when I spend all day at work wishing I was with Vivie (only to come home early and be too exhausted to be a good mum), I hate Stu and I hate myself more and I can't stop wondering when the real mum (my mum) is coming home to do my dinner-bath-and-bed routine and look after me – on those days I go for a 'quick lie down for five minutes'. And then I pretend I haven't noticed that outside my window it's gone dark. And I pretend I haven't noticed it's way past 8 p.m. and 'Oh my God, I didn't realise I'd been up here so long – I'm so sorry I left you doing all of Vivie's dinner, bath and bedtime, Stu.'

But I did, didn't I.

Mums will know that under no circumstances are you to ever, ever lie down, because once you lie down you cannot get up, because if you get up you have to go and be the wife and the mum and it's just too much right now, okay? So I lie there, in my bed of shame and regret, wondering what was the point in sacrificing a chunk of my much-needed salary to work part-time so I can rush home and be with Vivie when I'm not even with Vivie right now, I'm a deadbeat mum and a lazy wife in a Junkie Bed™. (A Junkie Bed™ is a term I coined. It means you sleep on the mattress and have a duvet without a cover when you've just put your bed sheets in the wash. Except by 'just' you mean three weeks ago and they're still damp and rotting in the dryer because you pretended that you forgot to hang them out and have just locked this fact away in your brain's filing cabinet to avoid it – so three weeks later you're still sleeping on your raw, period-blood-stained mattress.)

And I feel sick because I'm so tired from my job, too tired for my baby and it's not even fucking worth it because I chose a job that pays crumbs.

So what is it all for? I think.

I watch the flame waver.

And then I choose – every day – to believe it's for something. It's for Vivie, so maybe one day she'll think that her mum did something more important than make money, actually. Her mum made her whole job writing for mothers: the ones too tired to be mothers today, so they hide in their rooms pretending not to notice that it's gone dark outside; the ones knowing that someone else put their kids to bed so it's too late to go be a decent mum now anyway; the mums who lie there in shame. Her mum wrote for those mothers so that, maybe, if they could bring themselves to look out the window, they'd see it's dark – but there's a little candle out there, too. And sometimes that flame helps get those mums out of bed.

That's what gets me out of bed. That's what all this was for.

10 AUGUST 2023, 3:37 P.M.

Hannah: How are my ladies today?

Sinead: Yeah swell, just had my keyworker come for a home visit to see if today's the day I t-shirt gunned Viv off the balcony

Hannah: Omg did she ask again if you're sure you're doing enough eye-to-eye contact with her to enhance bonding?

Sinead: Yup, I said yes can confirm I have noted the eyeballs today

Hannah: Maybe it would be best if you got one of those signs they have in the toilets at Burger King where it's like 'Facilities last cleaned by Jimbo @ 3.20 p.m.' but it logs when you last made eye contact with your child.

Sinead: I will suggest this but I think it would utterly throw her as then she'd only have three other talking points on her literal checklist and we know she is incapable of winging it

Hannah: I of course am familiar with the set q's as they are unchanging, but I would like a transcription of today's full Q&A pls

Sinead:

T: Hmmmmm (smiles)

S: (smiles)

T: (smiles)

S: Would you like a cup of tea?

T: Oh no I'm fine thank you (smiles)

S: (smiles) So ...

T: [TALKING POINT ONE] How are you doing today?

S: Yeah, not great. Still not great physically too – I'm just so tired even though Stu's letting me sleep heaps. And weirdly I feel sick again, like vomiting and headaches. So, yeah, just not doing good. And like I know it can be normal that not all mums bond with their baby as soon as they're born but you know ... it's been a while now. And like I said at our last visit, it doesn't feel like it's changed. (I then start crying a bit) I still don't feel any attachment to her.

T: (Smiles and nods)

Hannah: Pause – brief sidebar pls. You told her you still don't feel any more connected to Vivie nor either one of her eyeballs, then started weeping, and she smiled and nodded?

Sinead: Yeah obvi. Every day this is her only response to anything. To give her credit it was maaaybe like a semi sympathetic smile? But a smile nonetheless – and of course the nod. The nod never leaves us. As sure as the sun will rise, the nods will be a'noddin. Anyway, cont:

S: Like, I'll definitely look after her of course – I'd look after any baby. I guess that's the point, she just feels like any random baby.

T: Mmmmm. You'll get there, it might just take time. And if not, there are groups you can join. But look at her, she's growing so beautifully!

S: Yeah she's doing great (smiles)

T: [TALKING POINT TWO] Now, as you know I do have to ask – are you having any thoughts of harming yourself or the baby?

S: No

T: (Puts an X through what I assume is the box labelled with these emojis: 💀👶🗡️😵🪦)

T: (smiles) Well that's good to hear, and you're doing wonderfully. And she's just gorgeous.

S: (smiles) Thanks

T: (smiles)

S: (smiles)

T: (smiles)

S: (smiles)

T: [TALKING POINT THREE] Oh my god and just look out there, look at that beautiful tableau of sunlight streaming in through the window. Aww, I can't think of a more gorgeous space to spend an afternoon, can you? The light in here, it must be so healing.

S: (smiles) For sure!

T: Okay, well I'll see you next week – you're doing great. And she really is growing beautifully! Must be all that sunlight (smiles)

S: (smiles) It must be. Thank you

Hannah: God it really is almost poetic how this maternal mental health service is such a spiritually full circle experience. In that the very nature of these visits is to prevent you from killing yourself and yet her visits propel you to do just that.

Sinead: It's incredible stuff ay. And she's right – this beautiful tableau of sunlight streaming in through the window will maketh the most heavenly backdrop as I t-shirt gun myself off the balcony and blast off towards the pearly gates.

The lucky ones

ON MINE AND VIVIE'S FIRST DAY OF SPACE CLASS – a baby sensory thing – the teacher told us about Mount Washmore. I have tried googling this to see if it's a concept that exists outside of Space class and to get background on it, but Google thinks I mean Mount Rushmore, so you'll have to just go with what I know of it.

The teacher explained that Mount Washmore means – particularly in the chaotic newborn days – you don't worry about doing washing and just let it pile up into a mountain so you can spend your days nursing your baby and having lovely contact naps on the couch.

Which is a divine concept, mwah, love, except what if you have two other children who need clean school uniforms and a husband who needs shirts for work? We're a family of five with three filthy children so if I don't do the laundry, we will have no clothes to wear. I appreciate the woman's well-meaning advice to just forget the chores, but I don't understand how Mount Washmore can work.

Also what if, like me, you suffer from crippling anxiety which is exacerbated by a filthy house, filthy clothes, a filthy bench and mess everywhere? I can only function – let alone rest on the couch – if my house is near-spotless with everything in its place.

For me, this was another piece of well-meaning advice that didn't coincide with mental wellbeing – I still haven't worked out how anything about motherhood does. A baby that clings to you all the time when you feel anxious and suffocated with too much physical contact? A baby that wails when you're incredibly sensitive to noise? Apparently, the sound of your own baby crying provokes a primal reaction sending you spinning into fight-or-flight mode. And now 'research is showing that responding to your crying baby protects them against future mental-health problems and negative reactions to stress' as it reduces the baby's cortisol level which, if left rocketing, can have long-term impacts.[24]

Fabulous.

Fabulous for both the babies, and the parents who already struggle with mental-health issues.

'A baby crying activates the circuits in the mother's brain that are similar to those that become overactive in people with obsessive-compulsive disorder,' says a Canadian professor at Yale University,[25] who has been studying brain imaging of mothers' responses to crying babies.

According to the study, which used MRI machines to measure stress response, breastfeeding mums and those who birthed vaginally are more sensitive and more triggered by their baby crying.

So, sucks for those mums – but don't worry C-section and formula-feeding mums, you don't miss out! None of the mums had pre-existing diagnoses of clinical depression, but they sure as shit presented with multiple symptoms of it if they tuned out their babies' wails.

We're meant to exercise, right, to be strong enough to lug our giant babies around and also for the oxytocin for our mental health. And I try, I really do. I have ClassPass, a monthly fitness membership where I can book anything from Pilates to Mums & Bubs bootcamp and yoga. Except I'm always running late for Mums & Bubs, and they lock the door if you're even one minute late. And I book into Pilates, but then I get tied up child-wrangling or tackling Mount Washmore so I have to late-cancel the class and my session gets deducted and I hate the class and myself and my clean-clothed children!

And we're meant to meditate, except I hate to and I really don't want to, thanks. If I have twenty minutes spare in my day, what actually helps me to zone out is rotting on TikTok, not 'listening' to a meditation where I will actually be running through my to-do list for the entire duration, and raging because the meditation is being drowned out by my whinging baby and my two boys shrieking as they slide head-first down our staircase.

And we're meant to sleep, because sleep is fundamental to both physical and mental wellbeing. Except at the end of an agonising 'shift' being both a mum and also a working mum who must tackle Mount Washmore, I need to reply to my friends' messages and book my ClassPass classes (which I won't make it to) and clean the kitchen and book Vivie's vaccines and pick my ingrown hairs and try to convince my husband we really need to have sex because it's April and we haven't since we were drunk at New Year's and I want to watch that show on Netflix because everyone's talking about it.

So if I do all of these things after 9 p.m., or even just two of them, it gets me to about 2 a.m. and I have to get up at 7 a.m. with the baby so that's five hours sleep max – except it's not, is it? It's about three hours, because I insist on rotting on TikTok some more and wondering if my baby has died in her sleep and registering domain names for one of my myriad Side Hustles that will never get off the ground.

And I'm actually lucky because when I got home from the psych ward, Stu took over Vivie's night wake-ups and feeds. He knew that getting a decent sleep was fundamental to preventing my dissociative episodes and for my PND recovery. But this joint decision wasn't without criticism, with one friend saying it wasn't right that I was making him get up in the night when he also had to get up in the morning to go to work.

Therein lies my gripe with mental illness stigma. If I had a physical health problem that required me to get as much sleep as possible, would anyone say anything? Why do we act like the brain isn't an organ in our body? Why do we act like mental illness is any different to a physical illness? And why do we laud dads as heroes when we don't do the same for mums who breastfeed all night while their partners sleep soundly?

And I still don't know how we're meant to do it all – even with sleep.

Sometimes my mind whirls when I can't sleep at night and I wonder how I ended up in the MBU.

How, when I was one of the lucky few deemed 'bad enough' to be let into the publicly funded mental-health system three years ago, and was still 'bad enough' to remain an outpatient three years later?

How, when, once I became pregnant, I was not just a patient of one, but two departments – Community Mental Health and Maternal Mental Health?

How, when I'd paid $8,000 for a premium, private Lead Maternity Carer (LMC), who by definition was responsible for not just my baby's care, but my care throughout pregnancy, labour, birth and six weeks postpartum?

I was so, so lucky to have all of those frameworks of care and support of professionals. And yet I still fell through the cracks.

Everyone seemed stretched and the only question I was asked over and over was whether I had thoughts of harming my baby. No, I didn't. But she was harming me. Or, rather, my experience of new motherhood was harming me.

According to Dr Felicia Low from the University of Auckland, potentially half of all women may experience some form of perinatal mental distress.[26] And many of these women don't seek help – not even from their family and friends. In New Zealand, suicide is the largest cause of maternal death, with a rate seven times higher than in the UK, where – according to a 2022 Treasury Maternal Mental Health Report – they allocate a significantly larger budget towards their maternal and perinatal mental-health system than we do.[27]

Eleven thousand women are estimated to experience perinatal depression and/or anxiety (PNDA) in New Zealand every year. Only 25 per cent of these women will have their symptoms deemed 'severe enough' to meet the Maternal Mental Health criteria for accessing help.[28]

So, to the other 8,250 women every year who have a baby either on the way or in their arms: 'Sorry to hear you're having a bit of a tough time – hang in there! But do let us know if you have thoughts of harming your baby.'

In some parts of New Zealand, it doesn't even matter if your symptoms are deemed 'severe enough' – there's no room at the inn. 'Oh, sorry to hear things have gotten worse now – and you say you are having intrusive thoughts and suicidal ideation? Okay, stay on the line, give me one sec. Oh, I see you live in Northland? I'm so sorry, we're at capacity and our budget won't allow us to take on any more patients. Hang in there!'

Consequences of untreated PND – aka 'hanging in there' – include broken relationships, isolation, increased chances of long-term depression and risk of psychosis. Studies have also shown that babies whose mothers suffer PND can have lasting psychological and behavioural issues.[29]

And even if you can get someone on the line and you tell them that you're trying to hang in there but it's all feeling really, really hard, hopefully what will happen is that the person on the other end of the line is someone like that nurse in the clink that I was lucky to be assigned. The one who saw I was a very sick girl who needed help, now.

Chances are, though, that's not what will happen when someone answers your call. Because in 2015, a Mothers Helpers Survey found 85 per cent of women with Perinatal Depression/Anxiety (PNDA) had experienced significant delays in diagnosis and treatment due to a lack of medical professional education and staggeringly low screening rates for PNDA.[30]

In 2019, Mothers Helpers repeated the survey and found only a small improvement in screening or education since the previous survey.[31]

Little had changed. And little has changed since. I'm just one mum, so I can't do it myself. But if I could change things even just a bit, this is what I'd start with:

1. I'd remind healthcare services that maternity care shouldn't just be about monitoring the baby's growth and development. While it's fantastic for a mum to learn her baby's head circumference is tracking right on average, how come no one's listening when she says she thinks maybe she isn't tracking right on average, and she thinks she doesn't really want this baby after all, and maybe she kind of wants to die?
2. I'd tell Birthcare to stop spending so much budget on HP cartridges to print Breast Is Best posters. Instead, they should print different brochures – specifically, something to give to the birthing parents' partner and friends and family. And the brochures should list every possible physical and emotional sign of PND, so partners know exactly what to look out for before the woman they love won't get out of bed anymore, won't hold her baby, and just stares out the window at nothing. They should be given out at every appointment long before then – in LMC waiting rooms and at antenatal class, and at Fertility Associates, before she's even a mum, in the hopes they'll read it and take a mental snapshot of how she is now and what her baseline state is, so when she is pregnant, if the tide starts to turn they'll see it straight away.
3. I'd find some money, somewhere, and put it towards quarterly compulsory education and training for maternal healthcare workers. So, if a mum is lucky enough to get through to someone on the phone, that person is not just listening to what she's saying, they're listening to what she's not saying.

Because a girl who is 'so charming, and so funny, with a lovely smile and jokes – an absolute pleasure to have here' only got one of the rare, priceless golden tickets in the clink because she's loud. This fills me with so much dread. What is happening to the mums we can't hear? The ones who can't laugh anymore, can't even smile, because they've been 'hanging in there' so long, and 'yeah I did call that number they gave me at Plunket but they seemed really busy. They did ask me if I'm having thoughts of harming the baby and I'm not so it's all good I'm probably just tired. Or it's the hormones.'

No one hears them, and no one sees them. And inside they're screaming.

I am Bono Corcoran Dye

WHEN I WAS AT UNIVERSITY, EACH FRIDAY I volunteered at Starship. While they wouldn't let me work with the kids who were terminally ill – because they worried it would be too hard on me after losing my mum to cancer a few months prior – I helped out with children who were staying in the hospital to have operations or other procedures done. I would spend my days making up little activity packs – kitted out with colouring books, crayons and stickers – or playing games with them to distract from where they were, and to give their parents a break to go get a terrible hospital cafeteria coffee.

When I was nine months pregnant, despite being on death's door, I put my limited shreds of energy into helping Paw Justice, an organisation that looks after neglected dogs in need. I would share these pups on Instagram to encourage people to donate or adopt – and spent the few afternoons I could get off the couch cooking chicken-and-rice meals for the malnourished dogs and driving out to West Auckland to drop them off. Stu was aghast that I was both up on my feet cooking when I could barely stand (and as

I've never cooked a meal for him in his life), and spending hundreds of dollars on organic chicken for random dogs when we eat meat that has stickers on it saying 'expiring tomorrow'.

Since becoming a mum, and particularly since battling PND, I'm now fully in my 'philanthropic era' – even more so than before.

During my stay in the clink, my husband's incredibly thoughtful colleague put an application in for us with Auckland charity Nappkin.[32] Founded by writer Hannah Norton, who lost her mum to suicide when she was only two, The Nappkin Charitable Trust is a sub-fund of the Perpetual Guardian Foundation. It helps struggling parents with children under eighteen months by providing funding for a night nanny for one night, so they can catch up on much-needed sleep.

Despite Nappkin traditionally only funding one night of nannying for mums in need, I later found out that Hannah had paid out of her own money for me to have three nights, because she knew I desperately needed it – and because she really cares about mums.

Emma, another mum Nappkin has helped, says her one night of proper sleep was 'life-changing' after four months of caring for her son – who was battling colic and screaming nine hours a night – rendered her a 'shell of a person'. Emma says it was the support of the nanny, who stayed in text contact for weeks after her overnight stay, that kept her afloat.

After sharing my own struggles with PND on social media, and getting to know Hannah more, I eventually went on to be appointed the ambassador of Nappkin.

'We couldn't be more stoked to have Sinead on board. In speaking about her own experience so candidly, she is paving the way for other mums not to be afraid to ask for help, making her the perfect fit for Nappkin,' Hannah wrote in the announcement.

Becoming Nappkin's ambassador was such an incredible honour, as it's a cause very close to my heart. If it wasn't for my husband's colleague and the generosity of Hannah arranging the night-help for me (okay and obvi my meds), I very well could have gone the way of Hannah's mum, and Vivie might not have her mum here today.

As time went on, my involvement with Nappkin increased, and I'm now co-running it with Hannah. I take care of all our communications and social media, and I oversee our public relations, as well as liaising with mums in need to link them up with nannies. And I urge them to always contact me if they want to talk to someone who will provide a safe space with no judgement, ever – especially when it comes to having intrusive thoughts that can make you feel like a monster.

We truly cannot underestimate the importance of sleep when it comes to physically or emotionally healing, and the idea that Nappkin and the work they do to help mums might save a life – well, I can't think of a bigger privilege than being part of that.

In the year that has passed since having Vivie and meeting Hannah, she has become one of my closest friends. We have gone on to promote Nappkin across national media and at private conferences, sharing our personal stories as well as the details of the work we're doing to help other mums. Following our interviews we tend to receive an influx of donations.

We recently brought in Hattie – my beloved sleep consultant and now dear friend – to provide pro bono sleep consultancy to mums, so they don't just get a night's sleep and then go back to square one. Instead, they have help and support moving forward.

We've also looped in a personal trainer, who specialises in women with mental-health issues, to offer workout classes to our mums. We know those endorphins are worth their weight in gold when it comes to both mental wellbeing and improving sleep.

If you're a new mum struggling mentally, there is a range of services available that can help you, including Nappkin. Please, please don't feel you have to grin and bear it. Having a new baby is no walk in the park, so if you feel like you're not coping and need extra support, please reach out to any of the following services:

Helplines

Lifeline 0800 543 354
Parent Help 0800 568 856
Need to Talk? 1737
PlunketLine 0800 933 922

Maternal Mental Health

https://nationalwomenshealth.adhb.govt.nz/our-services/maternity/specialty-and-complex-care/aronui-ora-maternal-mental-health-service/
Check what support services your district health board offers.

Mothers Helpers

https://mothershelpers.co.nz/
Offers maternal mental-health counselling sessions for those who have experienced birth trauma. Check out the PNDA recovery course Out of the Fog.

The Mental Health Foundation

https://mentalhealth.org.nz/
Provides information and links to support services.

Bellyful

https://bellyful.org.nz/
Nourishes and connects communities by cooking and delivering free meals to whānau with babies or young children who need support.

Parent Help

https://parenthelp.org.nz/
Provides free parent and whānau support in the form of advice, counselling and coaching.

Parent to Parent
https://parent2parent.org.nz/
A nationwide organisation that supports the families of babies, children, teens and adults with any type of disability or health impairment.

Mums4Mums
https://mums4mums.org.nz/
A charity that matches volunteer mums with those in need of a little extra help and reassurance.

Dayspring
https://dayspring.org.nz/
An Auckland-based charity that supports mums who have experienced severe PND or are living with an existing mental-health issue. Support includes counselling, home-based programmes to help strengthen the bond between mums and children, and classes.

Nurturing Families
https://nurturingfamilies.nz/
Provides assistance for families in crisis with items such as nappies, wipes, clothing, baby food, cots, car seats, prams, school bags and more.

3 a.m. secrets I will never tell your dad

- Sometimes when I take you for stomps around a department store I will not name for reasons that will become obvious, I give you a toy to play with. And sometimes I accidentally walk out and forget you're holding it and forget to pay.
- Even when you're not with me, I still always park in the 'mums with babies' carparks at the supermarket because I'm a terrible person.
- Every time I'm reading you a book, I skip pages because it's so boring and I want it to be over already – and you can't read yet so who cares?
- Sometimes I pick at the little dead skin bits on your head that all babies have. I am obsessive about it, pick pick picking the little flakes off even though you're not supposed to, and I think it's actually illegal.
- When I'm giving you a bath and Dad is around, I put on a baby bath playlist that has songs about splashy ducks. When

Dad isn't around, I play 'I Don't Mind' by Usher ft Juicy J, where he sings that he's okay with his partner being a stripper. I play this for you because it's a banger and also because I want to condition you to find a partner who supports any and all of your business ventures.

- One time when you were a baldy newborn, I used an app to Photoshop eyebrows on to you for an Instagram pic so you'd look better.

3 FEBRUARY 2023, 7:17 P.M.

(Three months pregnant)

Sinead: I keep telling Stu I'm not going to take this kid to Wriggle and Rhyme or whatever, it can come to Prego for burrata and Chilli margs.

Ruby: Don't be ridic, you'll be so into the bébé stuff when the time comes. You'll want to show off how much better your baby is than the others.

Sinead: No, I absolutely won't. Why would you spend your days at the zoo or Baby Sensory or whatever when you can just take them round Westfield while you shop? Baby classes are for people who have not one iota of a life.

Wanking at Baby Sensory class

POST THAT TEENY TINY BLIP OF PND, of course, I loved the first couple of months of maternity leave. We did it all, me and Viv: Space class, Baby Sensory, swimming lessons, walks to the French bakery. I forked out on annual passes for both SEA LIFE Kelly Tarlton's and Auckland Zoo, which I told Stu would be 'such a money saver 'cause we'll be there every week!'

All the mums would sit in a circle at Baby Sensory with our babies in our laps – mine looking utterly shell-shocked and in tears because she's sensitive to noise like me – singing and signing the corn song.

What is the corn song you ask?

It's a little ditty that extols the joy of the sun and the moon shining and beaming down on us. Lovely, lovely, wholesome lovely. But then we get to the next line which involves greeting the corn, marvelling at its strength and basking in the joy of it feeding us.

Yum, right? Who doesn't love corn? So juicy, a hero of the veg. Except when you get to this line in the song you have to mime the shape of a corncob. Which in practise looks like you're wanking a corncob off. And you must restrain yourself from sniggering and making eye contact with any of the other parents, because what if they're not thinking the same thing? (They are. They're also thinking, 'What happened to us? We used to be successful career women in our thirties, long-lunching with clients and commanding boardrooms. And now we are sitting in a circle wanking invisible corn.')

During one of the Baby Sensory classes I was so bored I decided to film Vivie lying on the floor as bubbles and streamers floated above her and while I billowed rainbow-covered scarves above her face. I later cut the video together with hectic drum and bass trance music and posted it with the caption 'cooked at Splore.'

In hindsight, tagging the Baby Sensory class was unnecessary and short-sighted as I don't think they were too pleased with this unsolicited ad.

Look, there are good things about these classes, don't get me wrong. Aside from the boring stuff like they're good for babies' development, blah blah blah, they do also give you a reason to get out of the house, they give you ideas for stuff to do with your baby at home that isn't just rotting in front of Ms. Rachel, and you might even make some new mum pals. But, if you are going to make pals, I must warn you that there are two types of mums at Baby Sensory: poodles and wolves.

My favourite writer and comedian Jessi Klein first presented this theory about women back in 2016. In her book, *You'll Grow Out of It*, Klein, who was at the time writing for *Saturday Night Live*, tells the story of when she and her colleague Emily were walking past the set of the show and saw Angelina Jolie sitting down to be interviewed by Larry King.[33]

Emily said, 'Isn't it amazing that we're the same species she is? It doesn't even feel like we are the same species.'

'I know,' said Jessi. 'It's like with dogs. A poodle and a wolf are both technically dogs but, based on appearances, it doesn't make any conceivable sense that they are, or ever were, related.'

They 'decided that some women are poodles and some are wolves. And no matter what a wolf does (makeup, g-string), it will still be a wolf, and no matter what a poodle does (sweatpants), it will always be a poodle.'

So, on arriving to Baby Sensory class, you must certainly not limit yourself to only befriending other wolves – you just must be prepared that there will be poodles there and they will, by no fault of their own, make you feel like a garbage rat. You are both wolf and garbage rat.

While you have likely Made An Effort to get out of your grubby pajamas and put on real jeans and a clean Cotton On jumper and mascara, I am also guessing those jeans may have a postpartum period stain in the crotch and your mascara both expired in 2019 and is also smudged into your tired ballsack under-eyes.

Poodle mums will be wearing stain-free jeans and cashmere sweaters. They will not have smudges under their ballsack eyes, so you will wonder where they get their lashes tinted. But they don't get their lashes tinted, they have naturally long and full lashes because their grandmothers are Italian.

And yes, this can and likely will make you wonder why you even bothered with jeans and mascara because no matter what you do you are a wolf. But you cannot let this dissuade you from befriending the poodles. I have many poodle friends who are both effortlessly beautiful but also great chat and very kind – you just must grin your rat teeth and bear the fact that, unlike them, under your (stained) clothes you will never be wearing matching Actual Lingerie. You will now and forevermore be wearing your size twenty-two Kmart maternity undies – and that's okay, because it's just who you are. You are a rat wolf.

I also have a friend who I immediately decided – upon meeting her for the first time – was a poodle. She had thick hair the colour of milk chocolate and a middle-parted sweeping fringe like an off-duty French model. She was wearing heeled ankle boots and long flared jeans which are now the fashion apparently – while I was still wearing saggy boyfriend jeans because I am not cool and also poor so cannot keep up with trends. Her skin was tight and supple but also plump with youth and somehow also very snatched?

Obviously, I was head over dirty sneakers in love at first sight, even asking our mutual friend for her last name so I could google her when I got home (but knowing she was too cool and effortlessly beautiful to ever be friends with a rat wolf). Months later when we had, in fact, become close friends, she would explain that she was in fact a wolf in poodle's clothing. She forks out a fortune on injectables, has hair extensions, and told me that 'everything the light touches' when it comes to her is Temu sponsored.

So, we cannot judge a wolf by its poodle dust jacket. And while, yes, wolves and poodles are different creatures, mums can and should befriend as many other mums as possible at these shit baby classes. I just feel it is my duty to prepare you for the fact that you will feel and look terrible in comparison to them. But how is that any different to anywhere else we go as women, right?

After a few sessions of Baby Sensory class and swimming and SEA LIFE Kelly Tarlton's, etc., I threw in the towel on all of it. I cancelled everything. I'm sorry, Vivie, if you're reading this one day – I wish I was a more selfless mother, and I'm sorry but it was all so fucking boring. There are only so many times you can wank a corn while your baby sleeps, and traipse around a zoo while your baby sleeps, and sing 'if you're happy and you know it, make a splash' in a pool while your baby tries to drink the piss-filled water and wonder why you didn't just do this for free at home in the bath – which at least only has one person (or maybe two, hehe) piss in it.

All of this stuff costs hundreds and hundreds of dollars for the pleasure of being bored to tears and feeling utterly degraded because you used to Be Somebody, actually, somebody with direct reports and non-elasticated work pants and a salary.

After cancelling all these things I did feel quite bad for Vivie –

maybe I was depriving her of stuff, or delaying her development. But then my Instagram friend Josie – a proper Early Childhood Education teacher (you must follow her on Instagram @playbasedpepi for so many parenting tips) – said that all those classes are kind of just marketing bullshit. That your baby gets enough sensory exposure from staring at the washing machine spin round and round, and that's free – minus the power bill obv. She said that babies are happy to just watch you cook dinner, or suck on the cat's tail, and that's doing the same thing as all those classes.

Josie reckons it's fine for me to just play with Vivie in our own minimally piss-filled bath because it's still getting her used to being in water and those swimming lessons weren't going to teach her to do backstroke right now anyway, and that we can pick them back up in a year or two and get her swim safe. It was lovely to try all that stuff out for Vivie. It's also okay to hit pause on it, at least for the first year, and pick it up later when they are actual sentient beings.

She says you actually have to do fuck all with a baby and they will still thrive, and that first year you can – and should, if you want to – save your pennies for stuff that's fun for both of you.

What is that stuff you ask? Well, I feel I've actually got two other genius, Dragons' Den-worthy, zillion-dollar-making business ideas. Do not steal them or I will hunt you down.

1. 'Friday after-work drinks' Baby Sensory class – but instead of being served stale biscuits (no, I don't want to join the baking roster, thank you!!) and cups of tea, there are wine bottles and cheese platters. And instead of sitting in a circle chanting 'Ba Ba Black Sheep' while wanting to stab yourself in the throat with one of the musical instruments, it's babies in front packs while mums gyrate to Drake.
2. Instead of Mums & Bubs screenings of Pixar movies or Suzy Cato, it's Mums & Bubs screenings of *Magic Mike*. The babies won't know what they're watching anyway so who cares? Plus, it's good to teach them about the gig economy while also supporting the arts.

Regardless of if you are currently expecting a child or have a new one or have an old one or have zero – if you take one thing from this book, it must be this:

In the words of Benjamin Franklin, 'time is money'. And what he meant was, who the fuck has any to spare. I personally am never not in the red and also, if you ever call me, you sadly will never hear my voice because I never answer the phone because it's Baycorp every time.

But you know who is not sad? Me and Ben are not sad. Because we both know that every spare minute you have in this life is precious. So, for the love of God, please don't pay $220 for an eight-week course of circle-jerking in a cold community centre.

Apps you need and apps you must delete

DOWNLOAD

Solid Starts

Tells you when and how to introduce new foods to your baby and what size to cut things into so they don't choke to death.

Roam With Kids

Costs $2 a month for a subscription but very much worth it IMO. Founded by a clever mum, it shows you what kid-friendly events are on around the city, which eateries you can drag shrieking toddlers to without being kicked out, which playgrounds are actually good and don't have those metal slides that burn your skin off in summer.

Tend
An online telehealth GP portal where you can see a doctor over Zoom and get prescriptions without having to drag your sick, miserable baby out in the cold and sit in a germy waiting room.

FACEinHOLE
An app where you can drop someone's face onto celebrities or memes. Why am I recommending this stupidity you ask? Because this will save you many times for a quite funny, makeshift birthday card for a friend when you have forgotten their birthday because you are a tired, brain-scrambled mum.

TikTok
Because you will not read a baby book, or any kind of book, for a very long time. Instead of reading or watching TV, because you're too tired to concentrate, but also instead of sleeping or doing anything productive, in fact, you will rot in front of TikTok until 2 a. m. most nights. And that is where you will get all your baby advice and developmental milestone education. Some days this will also be the only thing that brings you joy.

Temu
Say less.

The Wonder Weeks
The blurb for this app is 'Find out all about your baby's ten mental leaps. Learn and understand why your baby cries more during the fussy phase AND how you can support him to develop all his new skills!' I personally do not do any of the recommended activities with Vivie to support her developing all her new skills because I just can't be fucked, but it is a validating app to log on to for some random, meaningless explanation as to why your baby is being a dick this week. (It's because they are leaping! They are constantly

leaping from somewhere to somewhere and this somehow explains everything.)

Pond Koi Lite
I think this Japanese app was designed for cats to play with, but I somehow stumbled upon it one day and it is a godsend for babies. It's a virtual koi pond, with moving water, filled with fish and lily pads, and if you touch the fish they swim away. Your child and/or cat will be bewitched by it. Buy a second, second-hand phone to put it on though, because I refuse to give mine up to Vivie even for five minutes. I need my TikToks.

Uber Eats
Duh, for ordering wine to your door. My most-used app. Ninety-nine per cent of my screen time.

Manicare
Okay but first you need to buy the device that this app is for – the Manicare Magnifying Pore Vacuum. It looks exactly like a Satisfyer Pro. But it is not that. It is so much better, my friend. 'A rechargeable extraction device, using vacuum suction to remove debris from pores. The in-built 10x magnifying HD camera, combined with three levels of vacuum suction intensity, helps achieve instantly clearer, smoother and more luminous skin.' This is what maternity leave is for and what dreams are made of. Forget Baby Sensory class. Forget your friends. Simply connect the device to the app and spend your days in a constant orgasmic, transcendent state – glued to your phone screen and transfixed by your disgusting HD face gunk hurtling down a plastic nozzle, sucking all your sorrows away. Also elevates the 'picking cradle cap off baby's head' experience exponentially.

FaceApp
A must-have – use daily to photoshop eyebrows onto bald baby.

DELETE

ClassPass

You will not go to that hot yoga class, or the cycling one. You will 'accidentally' sleep through your alarm every day. Just accept that's who you are and move on.

Spotify

Just not worth the membership when you will never be able to listen to your own music ever again. The soundtrack to your life, now and likely for the next five years, will be Ms. Rachel's creepy husband, Mr. Aron, singing that grating song about ants sneezing because they encountered some pepper – all day, every day.

Airbnb

HAHAHAHAH you goin' nowhere fast, baby!

LinkedIn

Why does this app send us sixty-three notifications a day about strangers launching new start-ups and birthdays of strangers that we are not even LinkedIn friends with? Also, when you are at a Wriggle and Rhyme class singing 'Wheels on the Bus' and wishing to end your life, hearing about a colleague's promotion that you should have got – had you not been on maternity leave – will possibly be the final straw.

A sad beige baby

WHEN I WAS ABOUT TO TURN THREE, some vague 'aunt' (you know the ones, like a friend of a friend of your mum's hairdresser's god-daughter's person who does their colonics) bought me a birthday present. A special birthday outfit. But this was not just some basic bitch tutu and a sequin up and downy t-shirt that said 'Three! The bee's knees!' or something. Oh no, my friend! This. This was a fever dream.

A purple knee-length skirt – the exact same shade of purple as Barney the Dinosaur.

Oh, in cotton, you ask? Polyester? Oh no, my friend. This was something so rare, I don't know if it had ever been done before. This was Avant-Garde. This was Vogue.

A hand-knitted purple skirt, like an extraordinarily peculiar scarf to wrap yourself up in before stepping out for a brisk winter stroll.

And we would think, to offset such a statement piece we would pair this with a simple, crisp, classic white tee. Oh no, my friend!

Because this vague aunt, she was not afraid to mix and match colours, textures and prints. She knew that trends may fade, but style is forever.

The t-shirt was adorned with three cats. What's weird about that, you ask? Absolutely nothing. Except these were not pictures of cats that had been embroidered on. And these were not like iron-on decal cats, or part of the fabric design in any way.

These were three, life-size decapitated soft-toy cat heads that had been surgically removed and sewn on.

If I hadn't been three years old at the time, I think, to the naked eye, they would've appeared to be three hairy breasts with faces.

This outfit, it was the most stunning thing I'd ever laid my two eyes and three breasts on in my whole three years of life. To my parents' horror, I wore the outfit my entire birthday, from dawn to dusk. Then to their dismay, I insisted on wearing it to bed. And then (and I now think this distress may have actually caused my mother's eventual demise), I wore nothing but this outfit, every day, 365 days a year, for the next three years. It must have been manufactured by the same brand that made those *Sisterhood of the Travelling Pants* jeans that fit all four of those friends whose sizes ranged from 6–18.

Because by the hand of some witchcraft, this outfit grew as I grew. We grew as one. Those three dismembered cat heads and I, we became that disturbing 90s cartoon show *CatDog*, about the creature that is half cat and half dog fused together. It was impossible to distinguish where the cats ended and I began.

In a desperate attempt to separate the Siamese quads that were SinCats, every night under the cloak of darkness my parents would smuggle the outfit outside and bury it in the outdoor wheely bin. And when the sun rose, they would feign confusion and say they 'had no idea where that lovely outfit could be – I'm sorry darling that's so strange!'

And then after an extensive search through our property guided by my Elmo torch, I would find my beloved outfit buried in the bin, haul it out, brush the cigarette butts off the cats' faces and drag it back inside where it belonged. Hush now, my angels, you are safe.

And this three cats and mouse game with my parents would continue every day and every night. They would sneak the outfit out; I would drag it back in.

Until one day, after fighting such a long battle, the skirt breathed her last breath and simply unravelled. It seems there is only so much two-ply yarn from Spotlight can do to contain the now-rotund mid-section of a dumpy seven-year-old. Shortly after her passing, one of the cat heads fell off, leaving a hole in the t-shirt where she once lay. I had no choice but to make peace with the fact it was over – and I was, once more, alone. Fast forward to 2020 and it's no surprise I am scarred by the fashion of my childhood.

On my second date with Stu, he turned up wearing bootcut jeans and a shirt with flared frilly cuffs, so I made him go home and change. I know that sounds so mean, but I was already head over heels in love with him and desperate to keep it that way – so I really was trying to help.

The first time I was invited into his bedroom, I barged into his wardrobe and forced him to let me sort it into 'throw out' and 'keep' piles. Just twenty minutes later, there was nothing in the 'keep' pile.

I hauled every item he owned to a clothing bin, while he shrieked that some of those shirts (embroidered with cartoon fish on the cuffs?!) had just been bought a week earlier and still had tags on them.

I then forced him to give me his credit card, and I bought for him a capsule wardrobe of classic, age-appropriate but still cool basics – including a selection of plain, well-fitting t-shirts; linen button-downs; a navy knit sweater; straight leg Levis; a bomber jacket and RM Williams boots.

I made him go to the barber with a reference photo of Patrick Dempsey (obvi) at the height of *Grey's Anatomy* hair fame, and I made him grow a beard. I still show people the *Queer Eye*-worthy 'before and after' photos I made him pose for – and no one can ever believe it's the same man.

When Vivie was born, she would spend the first seven months of her life as a Sad Beige Baby – wearing nothing but bone-coloured onesies.

Sand. Ecru. Porridge dried to bowl that you left to soak in 2003 and 'probably still needs another minute'. Taupe. Tan. Your Spanx. Oat. Self-loathing (cottage cheese on rice cakes). Cream. Stone. Freya's Wrap.

Fawn. Ivory. Hummus. Clay. Almond. Flaccid penis eco-straws that disintegrate in your mouth because this is the cross we all must bear to protect small turtle nostrils.

Cat biscuits. Desert. Nude. The tote bag belonging to that one guy you dated who carried a tote bag (always either from Unity Books or Auckland Art Gallery to prove he is a Man of Depth. He is Read. He is smART. He is so cultured; he is those Yakult drinks. And he has not one single item in the tote bag).

Birch. Parchment. Self-acceptance (Wicked Wings). Camel. Oyster. All of your bras.

Your entire all-male executive team. Wheat. Sepia. The paper sheet you're lying on when the waxer asks 'back too?' and you shrug nonchalantly like 'I mean you can if you want, up to you, there's probably not much back there though?' and then you roll over and the paper sheet is stuck to your ass sweat and your shame and it's so, so wet and it rips.

Beige. Specifically, Beigey and The Babies (*sing to 'Bennie and The Jets').

'Sad Beige Baby' was a term coined in 2022 by TikTok hoot Hayley DeRoche.[34] It describes the visual aesthetic and booming microtrend of dressing one's child in head-to-toe 'neutrals' AKA as a tuberculosis-ridden – yet confusingly clean – Victorian orphan selling matches on a street corner for a handsome salary of sixpence annually.

In short – think Jamie Kay, Nature Baby, Kim Kardashian's house, Yeezys, North West's 'coloured ball-pit' (all the balls are white). North West's outfits. Stormi's outfits. And all the other Kardashian babies' outfits.

DeRoche hypothesizes that the Sad Beige Baby phenomenon markets the fantasy that 'if I buy neutrals, my children will also be neutral, calm and quiet.'[35]

While we obviously know it doesn't get more absolute wishful thinking than that, Dr. Leda Kaveh, a licensed clinical psychologist and director of Washington Psychological Wellness, sort of agrees. She says that 'if parents feel more comfortable with neutrals, it might create a more relaxed and peaceful environment for them, which can positively impact the baby as well.'[36]

Neutrals might actually provide some relief for parents who are collectively over their limit with the demands of parenting, which includes the unrelenting violent attack on the eyeballs by way of rainbow, sing-songing, jingly, jangly, flashing light, potential seizure-inducing plastic crap. And according to me, when for a huge chunk of that first year of your baby's life you have them strapped to your chest, it's utterly understandable that you would want a cohesive look, that shades of white and beige complement everything and that you don't want a small dog-sized Princess Elsa person belted atop your Anine Bing tee because then people can't see the Anine Bing logo so what was the point of spending twelve chillion dollars on it when it may as well be Kmart.

So, I didn't give a shit if her outfits weren't as stimulating as they should have been. Until I received one video from my husband when I was overseas for the first time and away from my child – one video that changed everything.

While I was in Melbourne for the Taylor Swift concert – a trip I thought I'd spend wracked with despair about being away from the baby, but I did very much survive as I am So Strong you know? – this message landed in my Facebook inbox.

A face-to-camera piece of Stu saying that he knew my biggest concern about leaving Vivie would be Stu not dressing her in my favourite brown colour palette.

Not to worry he said, panning the camera to her to the soundtrack of The Rolling Stones' 'She's a Rainbow'. She was dressed in fluorescent socks, stripy yellow pants we'd been gifted, her big brother's lime-green Minecraft t-shirt with floral bloomers on her head like a fortune teller's hat.

I shared the video, and it got hundreds of replies – the most I've ever had – saying all jokes aside, she'd never looked better. And I agreed. She looked fun, she looked sassy, and I realised how boring and washed-out she'd always looked in beige.

On returning home I sold her entire bleak wardrobe and replaced it all with fun-filled pieces, including candy-coloured vintage OshKosh dungarees, striped tees from the nineties that I sourced on Trade Me and pastel-checkered tracksuits. She now looks like a toddler from *Rugrats* who has microdosed acid.

However, I have not given up the beige entirely. While outsiders may see the neutral colours as limiting and dull, I think keeping to that colour scheme (see: Dulux palette the Great Depression) is a sign of freedom. That it's one example of a parent choosing to focus on their own needs instead of always supplanting them.

The Sad Beige Baby Moms dying on the sad dead-grass (beige) hill argue till they're beige in the face that the colourless colour palette is actually good for babies, as it avoids overstimulating them. They argue that babies are easily distracted and excited by toys, sounds, and colours and that placing them in beige rooms/padded cells may help them be calmer and more focused on learning and development.

As it's transpired, avoiding 'overstimulating' Vivie has become my entire life ethos – in that I've discovered it's the most divinely convenient way to avoid or get out of any and everything I don't want to do, i.e. being invited to a four-year-old's birthday party at indoor playground Popking, filled with 200 mucus-faced shrieking children and a piss-filled ball-pit? 'Gah I'm so sorry we can't make it, Vivie is just so sensitive to too much noise, crowds and bright lights.'

But being invited to an exclusive Friends & Family only Ruby sample sale in a jam-packed warehouse full of sweaty heaving bodies pawing through racks while you gasp for oxygen and choke out a blood-garbled 'no worries gal' when another Friend and/or Family elbows you in the face to get to the last pair of size 14 navy Firebird pants, smashing your two front teeth out? 'Should be absolutely fine! Will just strap her in the front pack, she's such a social baby she'll J'adore the hustle & bustle and the people watching.'

There's also an orchestra of beige harps harping on that wooden toys are more sustainable and better for the planet.

So, their argument is that lots of colourful baby items are made in unsustainable ways, crafted from harmful plastics, while neutral, wooden or beige items tend to be eco-friendlier and more sustainable. And that a lot of those plastic toys and colourful baby and child items also contain lots of toxins – so by eschewing such poisonous tatt, parents will expose their children to fewer harmful materials.

Which of course sounds very sensible in theory, but I think it's more likely that we believe neutral, wooden and beige items signal Wealth. And I perhaps think this too, because I regularly purchase one-dollar dupes of these designer boutique toys from Temu – despite being fully In The Know that they are likely formulated using the cancer-causing hexavalent chromium from *Erin Brockovich*. Because I want my home to look like Wealth.

Some White/Beige Walkers even insist that neutral colours and light wood are necessary for babies because they're 'the same colour as mom's skin'. So, the subtext of this messaging I'm assuming is 'if your skin is not as light/white as a $150 rattan laundry basket from Città, I'm so sorry but the outlook for your child is troubling to say the least – we're talking a one trillion per cent chance of Failure To Thrive – which can have devastating repercussions in later life, such as heroin addiction, becoming a "Girlboss" Arbonne rep and marrying a part-time DJ'.

So please, can we just call a beige sand-covered spade a spade? Which is that many millennial parents simply do not want to raise their children in the gaudy, Fisher-Price junk-filled homes – which were less Home & Garden and instead embodied the aesthetic of a grotty YMCA school holiday programme – that they grew up in.

Not because those toys were chemical laden or so over-stimulating that childhood aneurysm rates in the 90s aneurysm-ed through the roof, but because those toys were fucking ugly. And there is absolutely zero shame in not wanting a fucking ugly house and life.

Meanwhile, mark my words, I will not rest until I track down the condemned and cobweb-covered Dunedin factory which in 1995 produced a limited run capsule collection of cat-head garments for toddlers aged 18–24 months. I shall rebuild this factory from the ground up and we will re-release this archived range for every man, woman and child, and I shall be their Wonka.

What you actually need to buy when you're having a baby. (This is the only list that matters.)

- A Baby Brezza Formula Pro – which is a Nespresso-style formula dispenser. Yes, it's one trillion dollars, but it will save you hundreds of mind-numbing hours spent scoop, scoop, scooping five hundred scoops of formula into five hundred bottles.
- If you don't have a spare room, buy an inflatable mattress for the many nights you and your partner are not speaking to each other and don't want to sleep on the same continent, let alone bed.
- A breastfeeding pillow, even if you aren't breastfeeding. You will use it as a backrest to jam your baby into when they're

learning to sit up on their own, so they don't fall back and smash their brains on the hardwood floor.

- A hanging mobile for above the changing table. When they get to about nine months, your baby will not lie still enough to have their nappy changed and instead will flail around like a panicked fish reeled onto a boat. You must have some form of distraction jangling above their head to keep them still.
- Cask wine.
- Eighty socks for the baby: all the same colour, never any other colours. You will lose at least forty of them, so this way you will still have twenty passable pairs.
- A circle of neglect, AKA one of those heinous, garish coloured jumper things with tacky toys all over it that you can pop your baby into in the kitchen so you can get just one thing done, like make a single piece of toast. (This will be all you eat today, and every day.)
- A courier van full of rusks. Your child will consume ninety-three per day.
  — Crying baby? Rusk.
  — Happy baby? Rusk.
  — Bored baby? Rusk.
  — Tired baby? Rusk.
  — Hungry mum who does not have the strength to make that single piece of toast? Rusk.
- A baby bath. Not to bathe them in, but for everything else. Put paint in it for them to slither around in – it will keep them entertained for near forty-five mins. And when you CBF getting baby food on your floor, just give them dinner in there – like a literal pig in a trough.
- One pair of Lululemon leggings, two pairs of bike shorts, ten men's white t-shirts from Kmart in size XL, Crocs. This is all you will wear for the next year, nothing else. This is your capsule wardrobe.
- Tequila.

- A defensive driving course. Even if you got your driver's licence twenty years ago – in fact, especially if you did – driving with your child will now send you into a panic state and you will grip the steering wheel tight while clenching your teeth. You will be petrified of every other car on the road. You will become a Karen who calls the non-urgent police line once a week to screechingly report people for driving half a kilometre over the limit.
- Dry shampoo, fifty hair ties (because you will lose forty-nine of them by EOD), a little comb to do a middle part for some semblance of 'effort'. This greasy but chalky (from the dry shampoo) bun will be your hair for the next year. Just accept it.
- Also, one of those root cover-up-erer hair-colour-in-a-stick things to cover your postpartum bald spots.
- A little hair catcher thing for the shower because your partner will be both horrified and revolted when you use the hair that's fallen out to create little artistic shapes on the shower wall.
- Brown hair dye, because you will never again have four hours to sit in a chair getting a full head of blonde foils, even if you could afford it on maternity leave.
- A Satisfyer Pro because it is very unlikely you will be having sex for a very long time, even if you wanted to. Which you won't – no one does.
- Emergency cigarettes, if you're that way inclined. Or weed. And if my editor makes me take that out, CBD oil.
- Just one single razor. This will also last you until your child turns one, as you will no longer shave your body hair. Maybe armpits occasionally in summer, maybe one calf (you'll forget the other) if you're wearing a dress (which will be one time that year, on your birthday). Congratulations, you are now a feminist/chimpanzee.
- Couples counselling.

11 JULY 2024, 9:04 A.M.

Sinead: Hatts if I tell you something can you promise not to call Oranga Tamariki? Oh, actually wait maybe you should TBH, so just going to put it down in writing here for you to show the courts that 'my wishes are for Hattie Moleta to have custody of Genevieve Michele Dye'.

Sinead: Anyway, me and Stu are so fried right now trying to juggle all the kids and my book and our actual jobs etc. and yesterday it turns out we dropped one of the very small balls we were juggling because when I arrived home Stu sprinted up to the car with glee and flung open the door trilling 'Hellooooooo!'

Sinead: And I was like 'the fuck are you doing' and he was like 'what do you mean I'm getting Vivie out for you?' And I was like 'out of wherest?!! I don't have Vivie?! You were picking her up?' And Hatts, I think you can see where this is going because abandoned and rotting at daycare was wherest this orphan child was! May as well have been shoved in a fire station slot?

Hattie: Ahahahha STOP IT. She was in the best hands at daycare, that will not be the first time that's happened and it won't be the last time. We ALL have those days and those comms breakdowns with the other parent. Actually, I've done it heaps.

Sinead: OK thank you thank you. I don't believe you but thank you. Also, she absolutely was in the best hands at daycare. My hands are clearly hands that wave 'Tata Vivie! Out of sight out of mind!'

That's a shame

Things I haven't minded being mum-shamed about:

- Having Vivie sleep with a blanket in her cot (I did not know this was a Sudden Infant Death Syndrome (SIDS) risk – thank you for telling me, person on Instagram).
- Giving her a hunk of pumpkin to eat at five months old (I thought you kicked off baby-led weaning with proper food like a lamb chop, I did not know you're still meant to start with puree – thank you for telling me, person on Instagram).
- When her car seat straps were too tight and slipping off her shoulders (I didn't spot that, and also did not know you're meant to adjust them as your baby grows – thank you for telling me, person on Instagram).

Things I've been mum-shamed about that have really fucked me off:

- Having Vivie 'not sitting up straight enough' when I was feeding her (she was).
- When Vivie 'wasn't buckled into her Jolly Jumper properly'

(there are about eleven buckles. If one out of eleven is not done up it's very fine).

- Letting Vivie do 'messy play' and paint on paper on the floor, because the paint got on the floor (the paint is washable and comes off with one wipe of a cloth, so I do not care?).

The most irritating one of all? Being shamed for buying Costco or Farro meals for my family's dinner instead of cooking meals from scratch.

I have two kids, a baby, a husband who works, a writing job of my own which I do every spare minute of the day I have in-between wrangling said baby, and I've had this book to write?

So whenst should I cook a homemade roast from scratch? 3 a.m.? You're right, how silly of me to not take advantage of that lavish window of free time!! The laziest of bones!!

Also, many of these criticisms landed in my inbox shortly after I had only just come out the other side of postnatal depression, so my confidence in my parenting choices and abilities was already fragile. I felt attacked and deliberately shamed.

So, I have mixed feelings about what I consider mum-shaming. While I gladly appreciate any cautionary advice around my child's safety, particularly because I naively approached motherhood with a 'figure it out as I go along' strategy as opposed to doing a lot of research, I do think there's a lot be said for the delivery of this advice.

New mums – especially those in the throes of postnatal mental-health issues – and even experienced mums are doing their best. And I think new mums in particular – who are learning as they go, like it's their first day of school – should be handled with care, not obliterated for making mistakes or not knowing everything all the time.

I also sometimes wonder if (and this might be unfair) mums 'shame' other mums to make themselves look and feel like better mums. Yes, Vivie is my first baby, but she's my husband's third. And as I see my Instagram connections' children approach the age my stepsons were when I took them on as my own, I won't be giving them advice if I think they're fucking them up somehow. But maybe any mum with a social media presence opens themselves up for criticism, which likely sits at the core of what my husband thinks is an addiction to social media. Because like a slot machine junkie, I'm hooked on the high of the likes and affirmation of things I post.

When I had a bad bout of food poisoning recently, I posted a homemade, crafty playmat of activities I had made for my daughter in-between violent diarrhoea explosions, because I wanted people to tell me what an incredible mother I was – and I frequently post lovely things I do for the boys so that people tell me I'm the Best Stepmum Ever (!!).

I think I'm like a celebrity (except not at all) in that I want the Fame and Fortune of Success and none of the bad parts, like paparazzi (in my dreams people take pap photos of me). But like actual celebrities, I am occasionally slammed. After *Game of Thrones* actress Sophie Turner and singer Joe Jonas split, it was reported that the breakup happened because the actress 'likes to party' whereas the singer 'likes to stay at home,' and, 'in deciding to divorce, is taking "the best course of action for his girls"'.[37]

And yes, while she reportedly enjoyed wrap parties in the UK amid her divorce, she was also filming a movie at the time – AKA doing her job, which, in conjunction with her partners' earnings, afforded her family their lifestyle.

In 2023, Rhiannon Lucy Cosslett of *The Guardian* wrote that 'the misogynistic undercurrents of these reports are clear: Turner is an irresponsible, absent mother who has had the audacity to make childcare arrangements with her partner in order to work, and worse, attend a wrap party where cocktails – cocktails! – were freely available. Meanwhile, Jonas is a present, loving father who is going above and beyond for his children, and is choosing to divorce their mother, it is implied, for their own welfare.'

Fathers, and their choices, you will notice, tend not to face the same scrutiny as mothers. And while my husband does not post on social media ever, he is constantly verbally applauded for being 'an amazing dad, so hands-on,' particularly when it came to looking after our baby in the night.

Due to my pre-existing mental-health conditions, including a panic disorder, PTSD and Depersonalisation-derealisation disorder, I've always had very high sleep needs. I require at least ten to twelve hours of sleep a night to stave off dissociation episodes – which are triggered by lack of sleep, exhaustion, excessive noise, bright lights and stress.

After I was diagnosed with severe PND, for which I was hospitalised, it was necessary that my husband did the bulk of our daughter's night-feeds so that I could get better. Some fellow mums told me in no uncertain terms that it was 'fucked' that I was making – and letting – him take care of our child in the night when he had a job to get up for in the morning.

While I'm not denying how hard that was for Stu, if I had any sort of physical medical condition – and as I've mentioned in a previous chapter, the brain is an organ too – I doubt I would receive the same disbelief and shame around my husband supporting me. And of course, dads are never slammed for 'making' their partners do the night-feeds.

When I was pregnant, one of Stu's female colleagues retorted, 'Too posh to push, is she?' when he told her I was having an elective C-section.

Stunned, he reminded her that I was not only constantly vomiting with no relief and had both a broken foot and a protruding rib bone – which we thought would make contractions unbearable – but my dissociative disorder is also exacerbated by stress. So, we knew it would be incredibly likely I'd have a severe dissociative episode during birth, and severe ones for me last weeks, meaning I'd be basically off my face with a newborn.

Giving birth by Caesarean section, as opposed to 'natural' or vaginal delivery, has been a subject of popular debate for years. The term 'Too Posh to Push' began circulating in 1999 when Victoria

Beckham faced criticism after revealing that she chose to give birth to her first child via a C-section (she would go on to have C-sections for her next three children).

Oscar winner Kate Winslet initially obscured that she welcomed her eldest child, daughter Mia, via Caesarean in 2000. The *Titanic* actress didn't admit to it until four years later when she revealed she'd been 'traumatised' by not giving birth naturally.

'I've never talked about this. I've gone to great pains to cover it up. But Mia was an emergency C-section. I just said I had a natural birth because I was so completely traumatised by the fact that I hadn't given birth. I felt like a complete failure.'[38]

And, like me, Winslet is curvy and physically looks like she has the 'perfect' body to carry and birth a child naturally.

'My whole life, I'd been told I had great child-bearing hips,' she told the outlet. 'There's this thing amongst women in the world that if you can handle childbirth, you can handle anything. I had never handled childbirth and I felt like, in some way, I couldn't enter the "powerful women's club."'[39]

I made my choice and I stand by it, and my husband's colleague can fuck right off. I usually hate that 'women supporting women' Etsy merch crap, but all birth is birth – none of it's fun, in fact it's all terrible. So, let's all call a spade a terrible spade and no one's spade is less shit – we're all pissing our pants and hurting afterwards. No one's having a hoot.

When the late Peaches Geldof's baby, Astala, fell out of his pram, which she said was due to a large crack in the footpath, the photos were slapped across every tabloid around the world and critics claimed it was because she was distracted, talking on the phone.

But the fact of the matter is that it could have happened to any mum.

But – game-changer! – I figured out how to mum-shame without shame after one of my own many fuck-ups. It was the day I blitzed up porridge oats to make edible sand for Vivie (as I have a hatred of beach sand).

After I Insta-storied this, one of my old friends messaged saying she did the same thing with quinoa just a week earlier, left it out and it became infested with maggots. I was in hysterics that I'd potentially made a maggot nest for my daughter to play in, but I didn't feel mortified and shamed – because the way my friend had framed it was 'I did the same thing, you're not an idiot.'

So, I've decided that's how to mum-shame: just lie and say you've made the same fuck-up and we're all fucking it up all the time. Because when we're in something together, there's no reason to be ashamed.

And that's what we are, surely? A collective of mothers who are all learning and figuring out how to care for a baby as we go along – AKA complete and utter fuck-ups likely fucking up our kids in three or four mental and physical and permanent ways on any given day! And that is fine, I think! We are all crying shames!

Shame my name, shame my name! It is Shamead.

9 SEPTEMBER 2014, 11:22 A.M.

Em: How are things today?

Sinead: Well, I texted her on my way into the hospice yesterday saying 'I love you; I'll see you soon,' and she called me and was screaming that this is all my fault, and said 'don't ever fucking message me again you little bitch.'

Em: Shit. I'm so, so sorry. Please please try to remember that isn't your mum talking, it's the disease.

Sinead: Yeah, I know. I just felt like I was almost coping before that phone call. Now I just cry all day.

Sinead: But I still keep saying to her, 'I don't care what you forget, just don't forget I love you. And you do love me. And thank you so much for being my mum.'

But I think even that is pointless now.

Sunset

14 SEPTEMBER 2014, 12:30 A.M.

Sinead: Can you call me?

Em: Of course, my phone's on 10% will just grab charger, give me one sec

Sinead: Actually DW. I'm fine, I don't need to talk. Talk tmrw.

Em: Okay just let me know if you change your mind. I'll stay up tonight just in case. XX

Sinead: I just don't understand what's happening

Em: Want me to call?

Sinead: I don't know

Sinead: My mum died

Sinead: Why did she leave me Em

Sinead: I don't understand what is happening

Sinead: I just want my mum

Em: Sin, she didn't die, just her body shut down. Her spirit didn't die. She's still with us, we just can't get a physical response. Her soul will always be with us. Her spirit is right beside you now. She won't ever leave you

Sinead: People keep saying that.

Sinead: Em she loved me ay

Em: Sinead, she loved you more than anything else in the world. It's going to be fucking hard for a while – particularly this next week. But you're the strongest girl I know aside from your mother. Because Michy is a smart lady, she always knew life wasn't easy. That's why she built you so strong so this day wouldn't be so traumatic – and so you'll be even stronger for every day that's going to come after that. And if that's not love then I don't know what is honey x

14 SEPTEMBER 2024

@sineadcorcoran.dye has posted to Instagram 📍 Lake Tekapo

Ten years since my mum died so went to go see her, kind of.

I think she'd think it was so funny that I've been calling this trip the #deathtour 💀🚶🏔 because she was a lot like me and would lol all the time even in the most terrible times.

But I think she'd also be glad I'm letting myself be sad sometimes too. And she'd be so glad I get to go home to a good man and my own girl.

I put this photo here with Mum in the mountains to show her we're okay and to show her Vivie.

I know she won't see this post cause I am not a ghost believer and also I don't think ghosts are on the 'gram – but thought I'd post it anyway to remember that she was here and she is still kind of here and she is still my mum.

I don't know when the next time I come back here will be because to be honest it's been very, very hard.

And life is heavy enough – even for kids – so next time I go away I want to take my daughter too, and take her somewhere light and breezy – not somewhere where her mum feels heavy and might accidentally put her heavies on her.

But if I do come again one time, I might bring the book I wrote – and say hey I think you'd like this one. It's about you and Vivie and me.

My last will and testament

THIS IS THE LAST WILL AND TESTAMENT of me [SINEAD CORCORAN DYE]

of [Auckland] in New Zealand, [writer].

1. I HEREBY REVOKE all Wills and testamentary dispositions heretofore made by me and declare this to be my last Will and Testament.

2. I APPOINT [STUART DYE] and [HANNAH RORKE] (hereinafter referred to as 'my Trustees') to be the Executrixes/tors and Trustees of this Will.

3. I WISH to be cremated and for my ashes to be made into four signet rings for my husband, daughter and two stepsons.

4. I GIVE my jewellery to my daughter [GENEVIEVE MICHELE DYE].

DATED 01/08/2024 ______________________

MY LETTER OF WISHES

To My Executor, STUART DYE.

I, (SINEAD CORCORAN DYE), *wish to state my wishes in the event I become terminally ill.*

If and when I am admitted to a hospice – if someone well-meaningly tells my daughter [GENEVIEVE MICHELE DYE] *that if she doesn't spend every available waking minute with me in that dark, silent room while she still can – and not even zip home to her flat for a quick shower and a quicker beer on the deck and a lick of sun on her face – she will regret it for the rest of her life, I instruct you to tell her to ignore this advice, and that it is wrong.*

And that if she tries to stay awake all night and all day, eyes burning from sleep deprivation – because she'd never forgive herself if she missed even a minute with me when there were so few left, I instruct you to tell her to ignore this advice, and that it is wrong.

And that if she tries to camp out on a mattress on the floor of that room – both an island and a nightmare – to watch the bald woman, an unrecognisable and frightening shape that used to be her mum, who won't just die already – drag her out of that room. If you don't, she will chain herself to that island and that nightmare even though she can't breathe in there anymore and she's scared of the shape and all she can think is 'where is my mum to come pick me up and take me home?'

If and when I am admitted to the hospice, take my unrecognisable shape's phone. Nothing good will come of that phone now. Because that shape is not her mum anymore, and her mum is not on the other end of that phone. If on one of those afternoons in the room where she thinks she really might be suffocating now, she is brave enough to slip across the road to meet a friend for a quick beer – just for fifteen minutes – I might call her eight times. And she won't understand how it could be possible I am now using my phone when, for the past five days, I have basically been in a coma state, not speaking or opening my eyes.

You take that phone home because otherwise she might get eight texts from her phone network saying she has eight voicemails. And then, when about eight months after I die she is brave enough to listen to them – fearing the worst, that I was yelling at her for leaving to go to the pub – the voicemails will have expired. So she won't ever know what I said, and she will never, ever forgive herself. She will hate herself for leaving for fifteen minutes, hate herself for not answering the calls, hate herself for not being brave enough to listen to the voicemails sooner. But maybe even worse than that, she will hate me. For seemingly being in a coma for five days – not looking at her or speaking to her – until the tiny moment she took a tiny break for herself.

If my skin has turned from peach to a colour that will haunt her for the rest of her life, a peach gone so bad, a visual so disturbing she will never again be able to remember what I looked like before I got sick – you must drag her out of the room before she sees it. Because it is a visual that she will have weekly nightmares about for the rest of her life. Nightmares of an angry shape that she left so she could go to the pub. And in the nightmares the shape is yelling at her, and it's disgusted by her, because what kind of daughter leaves their dying mum to go have a beer.

And after you drag her out of that room, you call her flatmate and tell them to pick up a box of beers on the way home, and maybe a pack of darts. And you drop her home and tell her to go sit out on her deck and drink a beer or six; to tilt her cheek up so the sun lilts across her face, and have a ciggie. She might say to her flatmate, 'Mum would have wanted me to be doing this right now.' And her flatmate might say 'I know, I read that book too. Was she quite weird?' And she'll say, 'Yup!' And they'll both laugh.

And ten years after the date that I finally died, when the idea is floated of going on a family trip to visit my ashes – tell her that's not what her mum would have wanted. Because, otherwise, upon arriving at the airport to meet her family and board the plane, she'll slip on a suffocating clown mask that she won't take off until she returns home – and that won't be for days and days. And she'll spend the entire re-traumatising trip feeling like she must be the 'personality hire,' and make it fun and funny for everyone so they're not as re-traumatised as she is. And then she'll also try to turn her all-consuming nausea and panic about seeing my final resting place into fun Instagram content to cope, and will post silly selfies next to a snowman with a twig 'cigarette' in its mouth, captioning it RIP mum! *And then a stranger might message her and say that while she hoped this isn't overstepping, her pupils look concerningly dilated in the photo. And they will, because she might be taking so much Ritalin and diazepam to function that she will be constantly drenched in sweat with hands that won't stop shaking.*

So, you must tell her that on the ten-year anniversary, she doesn't have to try to make the day fun and funny because she's not the personality hire. She doesn't have to visit me, and I don't want her to. She can just be a girl who misses her mum.

Tell her to, instead, buy a box of beers and a pack of darts and sit on a deck in the sun and tilt her cheek up to it. And then tilt it back down, all the way until it rests on someone's shoulder. And if she still tries to put on the clown mask to try being fun and funny for that someone, make sure that whoever that someone is – and all the other someones in her life – make sure that they're someone who will gently take the mask out of her hands and say, 'oh no, we don't use these here.'

21 SEPTEMBER 2014

PUREWA CEMETERY AND CREMATORIUM

My mum told me once that when I was a little girl, I used to say to her that when I grew up I wanted to marry her, because I only wanted her and no one else.

I'm twenty-two now and I'm pretty certain I'm going to marry a boy, but in a way, I still feel the same. Because if I got to choose who I spent every day with, and who I got to keep forever, then I would have chosen her every time.

I know I'm lucky because I had my mum for twenty-two years, which is longer than both my stepdads and my stepbrother Cairo did. I know I'm lucky because for four years I've known that I probably wouldn't get to keep her forever, so I made every day count.

I know I'm lucky because I've got twenty-two years of memories with her. This year I spent my twenty-second birthday having a nap in my mum's bed with her, and that will always be my favourite birthday.

I told my mum every single day and every single night I loved her, and I know she never forgot it. Everyone always told my mum that I'm really strong and I'm really brave because she made me that way, and she never forgot that either.

I didn't get to keep my mum forever, but I got twenty-two years of forever. And she was perfect. I'm lucky I got to be her girl.

In the wrong hands

I LEFT WRITING THIS CHAPTER UNTIL NEAR THE END because I don't let myself think about my mum. When I do I often get sick.

I always used to see Instagram photos of new mums with captions like 'I literally wouldn't have survived this first week without my mum.' And I would think oh, grand news, thank you for letting me know my impending fate when the first week of having a newborn is finished.

But then I had Vivie, and I didn't die after the first week, and I didn't even really think about my mum or feel sad I didn't have her there to help me. She was not a 'mumsy' kind of mum and, anyway, it didn't matter that she wasn't here because I had Stu, and Stu was already a dad – so he had some experience with Mum Stuff.

Except now I'm thinking about her to write this book, which is making me sick and reminding me that it's exactly when I'm sick that I miss her the most. And in turn I'm reminded that during those long nine months of pregnancy, I cried every day because I just wanted my mum here to make me feel better.

When I was sick as a kid, she would put fresh sheets on my bed and fold the duvet corner down like a hotel bed. And I'd slither down under the duvet and she'd put her soft, ice-cold hands on my hot forehead and sing Edelweiss until I fell asleep.

And I know ice-cold hands is like 'sorry, what the fuck?' but don't knock it till you try it because it's like a cold flannel – except the flannel is your mum so it's the best flannel that swaddles your head so lovingly that it swaddles your sorrows away.

When she was sick, I used to tell her that when she did die, I was going to have her hands cut off and taxidermied so I could keep them forever and use them whenever I needed a cold flannel. And she said, 'That is a deeply disturbing plan but also really lovely, darling.'

I was her only baby, so when I was sick, she didn't have to look after anyone else. She could just stay with me the whole time – she had nowhere else to be.

But during those nine months, I had to wait in line until all the kids were in bed to get my turn to be looked after. And writing this now – because I've been thinking about her – I've been throwing up for hours. My stomach hurts and my head hurts. And I've had to wait for Stu to put all the kids to bed. But he's finally here now and he knows about the flannel hands.

But his hands are too warm.

So, he wets a real flannel for me – but it's not wet enough, and it's not cold enough, and it's not my mum or her hands and it's not the same, and I miss her.

7 FEBRUARY 2023, 2:34 P.M.

Sinead: Ok so when I went for 12 week scan. It was like clear as day and you could see the baby so well

Sinead: And Stu didn't film it! Like I wanted this for the gram. So today I asked him to film. And it's a blurry blob.

Chloe: Show

Sinead has sent a video.

Chloe: Just use that one heartbeat section

Sinead: God Stu. Like just do your one job

Chloe: Just like a 5 second clip of the baby with the heartbeat is good for insta

Chloe: Heartbeat audio is always a tear jerker tho

Sinead: That's what we want

Sinead: The money maker

The Vivfluencer

MY BEST FRIEND KATE REFERS TO HERSELF as 'chronically offline', meaning she checks her Facebook messages once a day, if that, and logs into Instagram once a week at the most.

By default, then, I am 'chronically online'. It's midday as I write this, and according to my phone's Screen Time tracker, I've been on my phone for three hours already today – most of that on TikTok and Instagram. And I don't just devour content, I post frenetically too. Never a day goes by where I don't upload Instagram stories – whether that's outfit photos, mum-fails or pieces of my writing.

I'm also disgustingly ashamed to admit that I had my phone clutched in my hand my entire wedding day and night, resharing Insta-stories in real time that my friends had tagged me in. I couldn't even wait until I got home, that's how much of a pathetic grip social media has on me. Even at our day-after lunch, I left halfway through under the guise of going home and changing out of my dress into a comfortable tracksuit – but really, it's because our wedding photographer had just sent us our album and I wanted to upload it immediately.

I became a journalist in my early twenties, and when I was asked to be Stuff's resident dating columnist and TV-show recapper, my online profile grew from the hundreds into the thousands.

I would spend the next decade documenting my personal life online by way of columns and on social media, and then became a very minor – maybe E-list, at most – celebrity as a video presenter. I also had a midday radio slot for New Zealand's biggest media corporation, NZME. I went on to co-host the official *Bachelorette* TV series podcast, and the followers grew again.

When I left media and had Vivie, I started sharing online the raw, often painful and debilitating struggles of being a new mum. The posts would often go semi-viral, and the followers grew so much I'd soon be signed to an influencer talent agency. Naturally, I started to post pics of Vivie too.

My line was that I'd never share photos of her in her nappy or naked, and never anything embarrassing – nothing that made fun of her. But I'd share cute snaps and videos, which would include funny clips of her eating a lamb rack bigger than her head, or kicking me in the face repeatedly, which I'd caption 'precious moments xoxo'.

Let's not forget that when Vivie was maybe thirty minutes old I was already cutting a sentimental video together of me holding her on my chest with a Taylor Swift song overlaid. They had barely stitched me up and I was clicking upload.

Over the months that followed, I started to experience a growing unease. Because I have a 'business' Instagram account, I'm able to access insights on my posts – which doesn't just show likes and follows, it shows shares.

Every time I'd post Vivie content, it would have lots of shares.

And while yes, I was choosing to post my daughter online to my 5,000+ followers, I naively felt like that was my community, I knew them in a way, and they knew me. But the idea that these photos and videos of my baby daughter were being shared – and that I didn't know why, or to whom, or what was the context of the share, it made me feel sick.

A 2018 report by the UK Children's Commissioner found that parents share about seventy-one photos and twenty-nine videos of their child every year on social media. On average, by the time the child is thirteen, parents have posted 1,300 photos and videos of them to social media.[40]

When I was thirteen, I box-dyed my hair the colour of a Sharpie pen and had a blunt full-frontal fringe that – despite the Sharing Shed charging a very reasonable $14 for trims – I would routinely trim myself with my dual-use nail scissors (the second half of that 'dual-use' was of course to trim my pubic hairs).

But because this was the height of the Bebo 'scene girl' era, I would trim it to rest precisely halfway up my eyeballs, to convey mystery, darkness and angst – all remarkably unfounded traits as a middle-class resident of the warm seaside village of St Heliers which had a non-existent crime rate. If you are having difficulty visualising my haircut, just conjure the image of the troubled young woman emerging from the television in *The Ring*.

As you know my mother tragically died when I was twenty-two. But if – by her hand – this 'look' was permanently documented on the worldwide web – her days would be numbered, and that number, Michele, would be zero.

The bio of a ten-year-old South Australian influencer named Ava Chanel reads 'model, cheerleader, dancer – DM for collabs, account run by mum.' She has 14,000 followers on Instagram and reportedly makes about $500 a month in brand deals.[41]

Her mum Zoe admits she has noticed a darker side to letting her child become an influencer. She has fielded sexually explicit comm-ents on feed posts as well as explicit images being sent via DM.

'The first time I ever received one I felt sick to my stomach,' she says.

She spends time every morning filtering comments and blocking users and has put safety measures in place to protect her daughter like not allowing her to catch the school bus or go to the local shops or parks alone.

She admits she is worried that a paedophile could potentially fixate on her daughter and has had lengthy conversations about the risks with her husband.

'We've gone through the pros and cons and had a chat with Ava as well ... At the end of the day, she loves it. As a parent, I think we are vigilant and aware at all times, but we keep going because social media is what she loves.'

It was a campaign by the Child Rescue Coalition that jolted me into a serious rethink about sharing photos of my daughter – the words 'vulnerable', 'paedophile' and 'predators' making me feel physically sick – and I started to question how much of her should be documented and readily available to all. For the first time, I found myself asking: why am I sharing? Who are these photos for? And more importantly, who could they be reaching?

Because once those photos are posted online, it's almost impossible to completely recall them – especially considering that screenshot and screen-recording features are now integrated aspects of iPhones.

Aside from the scary stuff, I've never been entirely comfortable with sharing Vivie on Instagram anyway, because I was sharing her life as if it was my own. And a big reason for that is because her father is incredibly private and hates social media. Nothing unnerves him more than a colleague catching him unawares and asking how the meal out he had had the night before was – because they'd seen it on my Instagram. He can't bear people knowing his business, particularly if he doesn't know they know his business. So, it's always been in the back of my mind worrying that while, yes, Vivie is half me – an oversharer who loves the internet – she's also half her dad. And what if she grows up and doesn't want to be all over social media, but it's too late and she never got a say in it?

A few months ago, after one too many shares of a photo of Vivie in Osh Kosh dungarees, I decided enough was enough. I wiped every photo and video of her off my account and cried. Because now when I look at my page – not only are the posts gone that really made a difference to people, like ones about the shame around C-sections, and the pressure to breastfeed – it looks like she was never there, and that I don't even have a daughter at all.

While I know that's a bit silly – of course she exists in real life – it still hurts when I document every other area of my life there. It felt like the final nail in the coffin of omitting my children from my life (I had never been allowed to share my stepsons either – both of their parents are sensibly also 'chronically offline').

I uploaded an Instagram story explaining that there would be no more photos of Vivie, and the reasons why. It hurt to share it.

I'm also angry and torn, because if I didn't have all these followers – followers I feel like I've earned through hard work, followers who support me and the work I do, thereby getting me more work and supporting my livelihood – then maybe my posts of Vivie wouldn't have been shared and I wouldn't have had to make this call to stop. I'm also gutted because I just want to be able to share my child's milestones with friends and family, like a normal person who doesn't have followers who are strangers.

One of my Instagram friends with a large following messaged me after I put the Instagram story up, saying she made the same decision to scrub her daughter from the internet after a woman she didn't know approached them at a playground and said, 'Hi Chloe!' to her four-year-old. Chloe's mum was terrified. She didn't know this woman and she said it frightened her that a complete stranger felt like she knew her child.

And that's how I felt every time someone from the internet recognised Vivie.

Even now, months after taking all the content down, I occasionally post something of Vivie without her face in it – like a video of her crawling for the first time. Again, that video got lots of shares, so now I'm wondering if nothing is safe, not even a carefully cropped clip.

Commander Helen Schneider, who runs the Australian Federal Police unit tasked with fighting child exploitation, isn't just worried about kids with big followings.

'My concerns, whether it's child influencers or anyone who is posting, is that you are undoubtedly placing yourself in a greater risk bracket… that offenders will obviously gravitate to users that are easy to access. What we're finding in the seizure of devices and the large amounts of data is, often, innoxious pictures of children, or non-sexualised photos of children, are caught up in this child abuse material.'[42]

I don't have a lot of photos of myself as a child. We moved around a lot when I was a kid, and my parents were divorced so I assume my father has some. Some might have been lost in one move or another, and I have the handful that were my mums. This little collection of photos – like all those of children of the nineties or earlier – are tucked away in shoeboxes and photo albums, away from the internet, away from potential harm.

For Mother's Day this year, Stu bought me a voucher for Milk Books, a company which makes luxe photo albums. We've put a note in our calendar for August 2nd, the day after Vivie turns one, and we're going to spend the evening over a bottle of wine, compiling all the snaps and all the milestones from her first year, of her and me and us.

And it will just be for her, and for me, and for us.

[I have temporarily reinstated Vivie on the 'gram solely to promote this book in order to sell copies in order to get some coins to feed her, so just a very temporary prioritisation of keeping her alive above preventing her being stalked.]

3 a.m. maternity leave Google searches

- Single mother benefit how to qualify
- Ms. Rachel net worth
- Baby ten months angry
- Is it normal that my baby has rage
- Should you let brothers fistfight to teach them conflict resolution skills
- Age calculator – how old is my baby
- Baby hair ties that don't snag
- Rat memes
- Baby ten months not crawling
- How to teach baby to crawl
- Baby not crawling are they paraplegic
- Can you take two Ritalin at once
- I took two Ritalin will I die
- Ritalin death
- Is Pedro Pascal single

- Is Pedro Pascal gay
- Celebrities who have married normal people
- Cheapest Botox Auckland
- Breastmilk still in one boob ten months postpartum
- Exercises to lift breasts
- Postpartum foot corns
- Postpartum sweat
- Postpartum snoring
- Can a baby choke on milk and die
- When will baby talk
- What to do if took too many laxatives
- Baby biting me
- Is Zach Braff hot
- Golden Girls old woman Halloween costume for baby
- Are burned pancakes carcinogenic for baby to eat
- Andrew Scott hot priest naked
- Toast size to give baby
- Will baby choke on toast
- Can you pop a blackhead on baby's cheek
- Popped baby's blackhead now scarred
- Do baby scars go away
- Best baby scar cream
- Where to buy alcohol miniatures on Good Friday
- Do Bloody Mary's cure hangovers
- What age can babies have halloumi
- When will my baby like me
- Baby ate peanuts watery eyes will baby die
- Baby feet so fat can't fit shoes
- Does my baby have foot lymphoedema

6 MAY 2024, 9:46 A.M.

Sinead: Hey Hattie

Not related to Vivie's sleep but um was just wondering – do you know if ten months old is a hard stage for some mums? I'm really struggling to get it all done and I'm not like ... enjoying her much? And playing with her is quite tiring and also boring a lot of the time. And of course, I love her, but ... I don't really like her much at the moment. God, I feel so ashamed, ignore me – please delete this text.

Sinead: PS So sorry for bothering you with this – I know this is absolutely not part of your job description and nothing whatsoever to do with sleep consulting!! I just don't have my own mum and when I met you, I thought you were so kind and idk, maybe might have some sage words of wizzy for this saddo.

Hattie: Hello my darling,

I am sending you lots of love, and hugs and strength right now ... here's my little novel for you:

Hattie: The first thing I'll say is that at ten months postpartum, with our first baby girl, I took her to our doctor for something like a cough, and I left with a prescription for antidepressants for myself. I had never felt that way before ... and haven't since. TEN MONTHS IS A REALLY HARD TIME ... I'd say it's the hardest.

You are the world's most AMAZING mum, no matter how you are feeling at present. AND you are putting waaaay too much pressure on yourself to feel a 'certain' way!! We have ALL felt like this. I don't care how much people paint a pretty picture ... the way you are feeling is 100% valid and normal. You are not supposed to 'love every moment', 'soak it all in', 'make every day a special one' that's simply not reality. No one feels like that every day. No one.

Hattie: It's bloody hard work, it's demanding, it's relentless and overwhelming ... and it's 24/7. We don't raise our babies in a village anymore, we don't have endless support around us, and we're expected to smile through it all. It's unrealistic and false. Please, please, never feel ashamed for not loving your time with Vivie. It is an unfair expectation for parents. It's a tough, demanding time – and it's totally normal to not love these days, and to feel how you're feeling right now.

And please don't let yourself feel any guilt whatsoever for needing some time away from her, and time to yourself. It is imperative mums have time out of the house and away from their baby. You will come back calmer, more accepting and refreshed because of it. This is SO necessary, and the mums I see fall apart the most are the mums who don't do this. They try and be martyrs and stay with their baby 100% of the time – this only exacerbates their inevitable feelings of resentment at some point.

Hattie: Vivie isn't moving yet so she gets bored easily. She needs you to fill that space for her and its exhausting. And you're right, what she wants from you is boring and unfulfilling.

You're doing everything right by letting her play on her own on her playmat, it's so important for her development. And when she's on the move she will start to entertain herself more, giving you that time back again – she's not far away from this!

Even the newborn days can seem easier than this, as we are swimming in neuropeptide oxytocin. I know your newborn days were not this way, but I want you to know how tough the 10-month mark is, and you're not alone. At 10 months, your reproductive system has come full circle and your hormones are almost back to their pre-pregnancy levels – this all contributes to how you're feeling darling.

Hattie: You still are, and always will be, an incredible mum who is honest, and fair, and beautiful inside and out. You will always adore your little girl, no matter what. But you don't have to love every moment, every day, every stage, every age, week, month! You just don't. And I can promise you that no one does.

Hattie: It breaks my heart to hear you're feeling sad. Please go easy on yourself sweet Sinead. You are making your lovely mum SO proud, every day.

Sending you so much love.

Call me any time.

Aunty Hatts xxx

Rate the pain from one to ten

SUNDAY 16 JUNE 2024 – A SNAPSHOT:

9:03 a.m.

Vivie is ten months old, and my peaceful, zen, chill baby has vanished and been replaced by a banshee.

After the Christchurch earthquakes, my grandmother, who we now suspect was bipolar, became convinced that her children and grandchildren had been taken over by body-snatchers. That we were no longer the real us, but something else – something evil.

I can't stop remembering this and having ridiculous, fleeting – but disturbing – thoughts of 'has that happened to my baby?'

Vivie frightens me. She puts me in a constant state of fight-or-flight, where every fibre in my body tells me to throw her down and run.

She is too big for the bouncer chair and it would slam to the floor if I put her in it – which I can't anyway because she'll somersault out. She does things like that when she is having her nappy changed or in my arms, and I'm constantly having to pin her down or throw my neck out from trying to restrain her so she doesn't faceplant into the tiles from a height.

When she's awake, Vivie just loves flopping around on the floor – so I can't look away for even a minute for fear of her smashing her head on something. She'll play with a toy for maybe forty-five seconds, then throw it down and grizzle.

When I hand her a rusk to nibble on – she eats about twenty-seven a day – she never says thank you. My logical brain knows a ten-month-old cannot say thank you. My other furious brain says 'why are you so rude?'

She's also just developed a new trait where she yells blood-curdling rage-yells whenever she's in the highchair, or in the car seat, or … well, anywhere. It makes me shake with anxiety. I feel like my brain is going to explode and I must grip onto something to stop me grabbing my keys and driving away from this family.

She won't cuddle me, she hates being kissed, and sometimes I wonder if it's because she's British like her father or if she really does just hate me.

When she does go down for naps – two hours feel like twelve minutes – I don't sleep. I don't eat. I don't shower. I lie on the couch crying, sending desperate messages to Hattie, asking if this is normal or if something's wrong with her – worse still, if something's wrong with me. I think that maybe I'm too weak to be a mother, that I don't have what it takes, that I don't have the compassion and patience a baby needs.

2 p.m.

It's time to wake her up from her nap. But I can't bring myself to. I'm scared of her. I pretend I haven't seen the clock.

2:30 p.m.

When Stu gets home from work, he'll ask me what time she woke and I'll have to lie and say 2 p.m. because otherwise he'll think I'm horrible and self-serving, that I put my peace before her sleep schedule.

I bite all my nails off until they bleed.

2:45 p.m.

I force myself to wake her, feet dragging as I slowly walk up the stairs. She smiles at me as I wake her up, because she is emotionally abusive. It must be a trick. I bring her downstairs and instead of reading her books and doing finger puppets like a good mum, I put her in front of Ms. Rachel.

I wonder if Ms. Rachel is the 2024 equivalent of a fire station, and we all consider leaving our babies outside her front door. Because she actually knows what she's doing. She does all the stuff you're supposed to do like singing songs and teaching them baby sign language – and she'd do a better job at being their mother than we are. I've started to withdraw from most of my mum friends because they seem to be doing better than me – they're softer and kinder and less triggered by anything and everything. Their babies seem to like them.

It's clear that what I really need to do is log into my office online HR portal and put in a request for two weeks holiday for some much-needed mental-health leave to clear my head and come back refreshed, in a better place. But there is no HR portal in this job that I paid a fortune on IVF to get. There are no public holidays, no long weekends – not even two-day weekends – and no sick days.

When Stu gets home from work, I throw the baby at him and go to my room, cursing both of them when I hear her giggling to him. Never me. I just get the yelling, the crying.

I put my hands over my ears so I can't hear either of them anymore.

I barely look at Vivie while her dad does the bedtime routine. She hates me anyway and I know that's what I deserve. He puts her to bed. And now when she wakes up tomorrow, she'll be one day older, so today is another day I've lost with her.

Another day I've been too angry to soak up every moment and love her properly and do a good job. I've fucked it all up once again. So, I beg Stu to wake her up and put her in our room so she can sleep next to me, and I can whisper in her ear that I'm sorry, I'm so sorry.

But he won't let her come into our room; he says she sleeps better in hers. A fair punishment for me.

I can't watch TV with Stu while he's able to zone out to a show and I can't. Instead, I sit here regretting every way I fucked up as a mother today, and undoubtedly will tomorrow.

I go to bed and take four sleeping pills to knock myself out. How else would I sleep, knowing what a failure I am and wondering if my daughter ever will like me?

And because I can't whisper 'sorry' to her, I whisper 'sorry' to all the mums I thought were exaggerating, or weak, or lazy.

I'm sorry I'm sorry I'm sorry. I didn't know.

I know now.

3 a.m. *Dragons' Den* invention ideas

- Kuber – Uber for kids driven by police-vetted nannies, who could drop the boys to karate and football in the evenings, so your dad doesn't have to abandon me during witching hour.
- A hamster-style water bottle feeding-spout thing but it's a bottle of formula hooked onto the side of your crib so I don't have to crane over in the middle of the night, splintering my spine into smithereens.
- Duolingo but for baby crying so I know what your problem is, please.
- Jackets that compress and go flat so I can still fit you in your car seat in winter.
- Silicone baby plates that can tell the difference between a baby trying to rip it off the table and fling food around and a parent cleaning up after, because trying to prise that thing off the bench makes me feel like I'm going to have an aneurysm.

Guilty as sin

I DON'T REMEMBER IF I WAS IN CHILDCARE as a baby or toddler, and my mum is dead so I can't check. But I know as the primary schooler of a single mum, I needed to be in after-school care so she could work enough to pay the rent.

I understood at the time – and, of course, I understand now – that she had to work late. But I also remember that I missed her, all the time. Probably just as much as I miss her now. Which is why I always thought that, when I had children, I'd want to stay home with them until they went to school – if I had the privilege to – and never put them into any sort of childcare. I also decided very early on that I would have a job that allowed me to work from home, so that I could be with them in the mornings and after school and never miss an athletics day or school production. And up until Vivie turned nine months old, that was still the plan. But somewhere along the way I changed my mind – and I feel sick about it.

I used to feel sorry for the other mums in my antenatal group whose maternity leave was running out and who had to go back to full-time work.

Now I envy them.

By ten months, Vivie had entered a phase where she could say a few words, but she was the only baby left in our group who couldn't crawl, while some of the others were walking. Everyone says she's grizzly and frustrated because she desperately wants to be able to move herself, so I'm trying to be empathetic, but her apparent frustration makes me very anxious.

Every phase before this one has felt comparatively easy. Literally as soon as I got home from Starship, discharged with a stack of meds to combat my PND, I logged into my laptop and relaunched my freelance writing business. While I didn't love the fact I was having to work while simultaneously caring for a newborn (because we were so financially destroyed after I'd had to leave my job due to my dissociative disorder, prior to the pregnancy), it was piss easy.

Vivie would snooze on a bouncer next to me, while I tapped away and was able to put loads of washing on, make myself lunch and post silly crap on Instagram. Now she's ten months and I can't do anything easily.

She'll sit on her mat and play with a toy for about three minutes max before she starts crying because she's over it. And while I understand, because I would not be riveted by rolling a plastic ball either, I'm also so over it.

I love her obviously, but this age is so hard. She's annoying and exhausting and I want to be anywhere but here – but when I do palm her off to someone else, I feel physically sick with guilt because this wasn't the plan, and aren't I meant to be soaking up every moment because the days go slow, but the years go fast, or whatever?

But there's only about three moments a week right now that I want to soak up. The rest I am struggling through, and I hate that I'm struggling. I want to hang out with her, but she's very boring right now, and she doesn't say much beyond this creepy screeching-ghost sound that makes her face go red to the point where it looks like her head is going to explode.

(I'm sorry, Vivie, if one day you're reading this, but I think it's a season, and this season you are quite crap.)

In theory, it's so easy to say that mums need a break to recharge and refill their cups so they come back to their kid more refreshed, etc., but in practice it doesn't make the guilt any easier.

As I write this, Vivie's at a friend's place. I've put an hour aside to work and then I'm going to Pilates, and while I know both things are good to get done, somehow it doesn't feel right. Why do I feel like a cop-out of a mother and wracked with guilt?

I've been scouting daycares for the past few months (I've done all the scouting of course, because mums do everything admin-y when it comes to kids, right?) but the good ones have a three-day minimum per week, which both my guilt and my wallet would not allow.

The bad ones are terrifying.

One that I visited claimed a 1:4 teacher-to-baby ratio, but when I went into the baby room there were two teachers to about twelve babies – and one of those teachers looked about fourteen years old and stoned.

It looked like two-thirds of the babies had cuts and/or bruises on their faces and, while I get that kids get rough-and-tumbled during playtime, it was too high a battered-face ratio for me.

When I asked one of the teachers what the babies were fed for lunch, she proudly replied, 'Carrot sandwiches or lentil soup, because it's cheap to make.'

The frugal reasoning of Oliver Twist-esque lentil gruel is not even what disturbed me. I was just utterly obsessed with figuring out what form the carrot would take between two slices of bread – which Vivie can't even eat as she doesn't have molars yet. Was it chunks? Grated? Julienned?

We shall never know, as I sprinted out of there shouting, 'Thanks we loved it! We shall be in touch!' over my shaking shoulders, Vivie tucked under an armpit like a football never to return to that field.

After putting a plea on Instagram for recommendations for a flexible daycare option with non-orphanage vibes, where I could drop Vivie off for just a couple of hours here and there, I got a tip from a fellow mum whose child went to an in-home childcare situation in a nearby suburb. While the logistics were perfect for what I was after, all I could imagine was (very niche reference incoming) that scene in the early-90s Mary-Kate and Ashley flick *It Takes Two*, when one of them is dropped off at a foster home where two unhinged parents fling the kids into the backyard-cum-junkyard to work on bits of steel.

My fears around daycares are also derived from my TikTok feed serving me countless news videos about children who have died at kindies through accidents or not being supervised. Friends are constantly telling me to delete TikTok, which is very sensible, because even when I was pregnant I would search for videos of C-section complications and then not be able to sleep (surprise!). But of course, I shall ignore their advice because I am rotten and addicted.

Earlier this month Vivie spent her first 'day' (three and a half hours) at the in-home childcare centre, even though I had no work on. I say 'even though' because after I dropped her off – and she cried – I sat in my car outside and I felt ill that I'd put my tiny (huge) baby in a daycare just to have some Me Time. I judged myself like I secretly judge my friend whose children are in daycare full-time even though she spends her days working out and watching TV. I took myself out to lunch to celebrate not taking a clonazepam to dull my guilt, then got a pedicure, went op-shopping and got a frozen yoghurt. I joked on Instagram that I was living like it was my last day before getting the chair.

A day later Vivie was sick with a virus and gastro – as is the way with daycare and with two older brothers at school who bring home every bug going. She's had COVID twice and scarlet fever once, and she's not even one.

Plunket and other parents tell me it's going to be great for her immunity long-term, but also shut up because I'm the one who is constantly short-term trapped at home with a diarrhoea-ing baby.

Our nanny – who comes on Mondays – is the world's worst nanny. She chatters to me incessantly about absolutely nothing, which utterly defeats the purpose of her being there. Also, I am at least forty minutes late to every meeting or appointment because she simply must know what I think of these hair clips she's found on Shein and also where do I think she should get her hair done? And what should she get done? And also have I ever tried clip-on hair, and speaking of hair her son is coming up for Easter and was I aware that in the *Mamma Mia* sequel (Here We Go Again!) the iconic 'Dancing Queen' scene, where the young and old Donna sing and dance together, was actually filmed on the same day for both the younger and older versions of the character? And interestingly (!!!) Meryl Streep's hair isn't naturally curly; she wore a wig for the role and have I ever tried clip-on hair?

Our nanny – who comes on Mondays – is the world's best nanny. She is sing-songy but very softly spoken, like a perfectly sedated Ms. Rachel. She is a weighted blanket in human form – weighing exactly one kilogram – which is also perfectly perfect because à la Sleep Foundation recommendations for optimal comfort this is ten per cent of Vivie's body weight.

When she is with us, she is never not wearing an enraptured Vivie as a lovely warm scarf nestled into her neck.

And when she is not with us, we are never not with her. Because when she next comes back to us, it's bearing painstakingly hand-sewn clothes for Vivie, a vintage baby doll cot she hunted TradeMe for and then sanded down and repainted in a non-offensive colour, or her very own baby doll.

Except it's not a doll. Because apparently one time I mentioned I liked that little white kitten Marie from the 1970s Disney cartoon *The Aristocats* because of her 'slutty little come-hither vibe'. So instead, the doll is a painstakingly hand-sewn cat made of cloth – but appropriately and devastatingly reimagined with little button eyes.

This year was my first Mother's Day as a 'real' mum. But this year was my fourth year of getting Mother's Day gifts - because she always reminds the boys to get or make me something. And by reminds, I mean forces – I assume by waiting until they go to sleep before gently and legally gripping their limp slumbering hands around a crayon to scrawl 'we love you Sinead'.

And for the first time in years, I discovered there was, in fact, something she had not made me violently aware of.

That if - upon starting a new nanny role with a new family - she learns the mum is battling PND, the next time she comes she'll bring a book. Not for the mum, but for the partner, and she tells them that for the next year, whenever they can, they should quietly take photos of the mum when she's with the baby, and put these photos into the book.

So that one day when that mum is beating herself up because she was 'barely there that first year', it might just be for one day. Because he can pull out the book and show her she was there the whole time, and even though the mum might not remember it like that…

'See that baby in the photo next to you, that smile? Look who they're looking at.'

And, no shit, she of course does all that Baby Sensory, messy play stuff that I did for about three days and gave up because I couldn't be bothered with the cleanup – and because I was also traumatised by my last attempt.

After pulling Vivie out of Monday Baby Sensory class because, like me, she seems very sensitive to noise and would shake in distress at the music and ten other babies' racket, I organised a miniature weekly sensory class with my antenatal mum friends and their four babies.

I offered to host the first one and decided to make a huge batch of jelly (Weight Watchers sugar-free in case the babies ate it – see, I put a lot of effort and thought into this) for them all to play in.

When it came time for the 'class', it was a freezing autumn day, but we said, 'no matter – they'll warm up in the jelly!' We got the babies naked and put them in a plastic bath on the deck and I dumped the vat of jelly on their heads.

I honestly don't know what I was thinking. Was I Joe Rogan hosting an episode of *Fear Factor*? Was the head-dumping absolutely necessary?

The babies turned blue and let out blood-curdling screams, which I thought was quite dramatic guys – it's just some lovely jelly?! But then I put my hand in it, and it was the temperature of the sea into which the Titanic passengers plunged.

We flung the babies into a warm shower, and we never held a sensory class again.

So, we shall daycare and have nannies. I've decided that what's best for both of us is better quality time, not bigger quantity time. If you love something let it go, etc., so please let me go away for a bit, Vivie, even though I feel shit about it a lot of the time.

At the time of writing, I've just had a job interview for a part-time role, twenty-two hours a week, which I feel will be a good balance between being with Vivie and being away from her to earn money that we so desperately need to get out debt. But a few months ago, I came up with another genius, million-dollar idea to appease parent-guilt (so please don't steal it because I really want to develop this and become a big fancy entrepreneur with no money worries).

It's a sleepy stories app for parents, but instead of Matthew McConaughey voicing a tale of the mysteries of the universe in his treacly, dulcet tones, I want to use AI to generate a customised story, using input from that day's caregivers about all the great things the child did that day at school or in daycare. Then, when the parents go to bed that night, they can listen to the story as they drift off, hearing all about how Vivie had a lovely time building sandcastles with her nanny, playing her xylophone and learning 'Ring-a-Ring o' Roses', and not freezing to death by the hand of iceberg jelly.

(I might still try to get McConaughey involved, actually.)

1 AUGUST 2024

Dear Vivie

Today you are one!

I cried the other day listening to a Taylor Swift song. I think the song is about a mean guy, but it made me think of you. You've touched every part of me.

I picked this card because you love dogs licking your face. And you love crackers, bananas, toy bunnies, Ms. Rachel, frights from your brothers, being chased, when I shout 'BODY-SLAM!!' and body-slam you onto the bed (but like gently obv) and baths with me.

I used to like heaps of stuff. But none of it is anything to me now, 'cause I like you the best. You are the making of me. You get better every day.

I'll put this card somewhere safe so when you learn how to read you can read it whenever you like, and know you were the best thing I ever did.

I hope this year you learn how to kiss back LOL but it's OK if you don't, I'll keep kissing ya either way.

Happy birthday baba.

Love, Mum xx

A tiny, curated selection of all the things I feel guilty about

- I have never taken Vivie to the beach – not even once – or anywhere with a sandpit, because I hate sand and don't want it in my car.
- Once when she was tiny, I used a credit card to squeeze a blackhead on her face and it left a scar.
- She loves having baths with me and I hate it, but I do it for six minutes max and only so I can get a cute photo of us for Instagram.
- She was three months old last Halloween, and I put her in a synthetic chicken costume from Temu that she was roasting to death in, but I wouldn't take her out until I got a cute photo for Instagram.
- I broke the carry basket on her pram by putting three bottles of wine in it.

- When I'm anxious (and under the guise of it being a 'bonding activity' that she loves), I put Vivie on my lap and use tweezers to gently peel off flakes of her cradle cap, then methodically comb them out, because it sends me into a transcendental trance.
- I often put her down for a nap an hour early and leave her sleeping an hour late because I want to watch TikToks.
- I put her hair in cute ponytails, even though I know the hair ties snag her.
- I don't let her eat fish for dinner, despite the fact she loves it, because I can never get the smell off my hands.
- Sometimes when other lovely mums give me lovely hand-me-down clothes that I hate, I throw them in a clothing bin.
- I secretly love when Vivie gets sick because it's the only time she's clingy and wants to cuddle with me. So I'm basically Gypsy Rose Blanchard's mum, and might have Munchausen by Proxy.
- When Stu does her bedtime routine, he reads three books and sings 'Twinkle Twinkle Little Star' twice. When I do her bedtime routine, I put her in her cot and say 'nuh-night, bye' and run away.
- When I come home from work and see Stu's inside with all the kids, I park down the street and sit in my car for thirty minutes recording myself singing (to check if I can sing) and also picking my scalp dermatitis.
- On occasions when I've been hungover, Vivie has watched Ms. Rachel for eight hours straight, from sunrise to sunset.
- Barring just a few normal adult-person meals, all I have eaten through the duration of writing this book – and this is genuinely not an exaggeration – is peanut butter sandwiches (don't have emotional strength to wait for bread to toast) and bowls of granola in my home office. And by home office I mean Junkie Bed™, which now features dried-out granola chunks embedded in the mattress under my spine.
- On two occasions when I've had to run into the dairy and

haven't had the energy to get Vivie in and out of her car seat, I've asked random roadworkers to keep an eye on her.

- When I can't be bothered going to social engagements, I say I'm stuck at home with the baby even though I'm just going to film myself doing dance routines to check if I can dance and also pick at my scalp dermatitis.
- I chose to become a journalist earning about $3 annually, and married an editor who, thank God, is much more senior than me so earns $4.50 – so Vivie, in theory, would stand to inherit $75 except, of course, I spent it on Temu toupees to cover my nine significant bald patches from picking my scalp dermatitis, and now instead of $75, she will be the heiress of a toupee collection.
- I have to be away from her all the time to earn my $3 annually, and it doesn't even feel worth it, because it's not like I'm a surgeon making heaps of money to bring home. And even if I was, I don't think any amount of money would take away the constant nausea and heartache that smacks me sideways with a lead pipe every morning that I walk out the door.
- One time I had to call the Poisons Centre because she ate one of my anxiety pills that had fallen on the floor – and by one time, I mean three times.
- Sometimes when I come home from work and Stu has been with Vivie all day I still say, 'Argh so sorry, I have to go upstairs to finish off some work,' and I lie on my bedroom floor watching *Britain's Got Talent* Golden Buzzer auditions on YouTube.
- Last Friday I put Vivie into daycare for five hours so I could finish this book and instead I lay on the couch using Photoshop to turn a photo of her into a Pokémon.
- I think I was a really cold, self-serving stepmum before I became a mum and learned that kids are just kids and I am not the main character.
- Sometimes, when I don't have the time or willpower to cook

Vivie porridge and spoonfeed it to her, I give her twelve tiny cookies on a plate for breakfast, like a dog with kibble.

- I used to care that me and Stu weren't having sex and now I don't care one iota.
- When I buy something online (which is thrice a day), I tell Stu it cost about $40 and he says, 'Sinead, we don't have $40 to just throw around,' but it actually cost $80 (except it didn't, it cost $130).
- I smuggle these online purchases into the house in my handbag, and at night-time under the cloak of darkness I shove the wrapping down to the bottom of the neighbour's outdoor wheelie bin.
- I have a saved watchlist of rental properties that I examine weekly, and contemplate leaving for.
- I applied for the single-mother benefit in preparation for my New Life, then realised the pittance would not cover rent on the most depressing, ugly studio flat you've ever seen, so how would I buy stuff off Temu AKA get any joy in my life? – so I haven't left yet.
- I don't give one single fuck about my career or climbing the corporate ladder anymore, and I don't want to 'have it all.' My feminist hero is not Gloria Steinem or Malala, it's Ali Wong. Specifically, when she said, 'I don't want to work anymore. I don't want to lean in, okay? I want to lie down. I want to lie the fuck down. I think feminism is the worst thing that ever happened to women—our job used to be no job. We had it so good!' I want to be a stay-at-home Trad Wife. Except not cook or clean, just, like, stay at the home.
- Vivie just turned one and it's the end of the book soon and I've only just started to really, truly, love her.
- Sometimes I wish I could go back to when I didn't really know her yet and didn't really love her yet. Because that was less scary than having my whole life in one little girl out there in a world where I can't always keep her safe.

A picture book for Vivie

I DON'T WANT TO WAIT till Vivie is grown up and can 'handle' finding out about my mental-health issues. I want her to grow up knowing and understanding that while Mum is okay most of the time – some days Mum isn't. But it's okay, because Mum can usually get better all on her own. Even if she has to go away for a little bit, she always thinks Vivie is great – that never changes. I want her to learn that, just like how sometimes we're too sick to go to our work-jobs, sometimes mums are too sick to go to their mum-jobs (even though they want to) and that's okay – and normal.

A while ago, I hunted around on Google for kids' books that explain a parent's mental illness in an age-appropriate, digestible and non-terrifying fashion, but I struggled to find anything for kids under nine, and the majority of them were about borderline personality disorder and bipolar. So, as I want to start reading these books to her now (early bird catches the generational trauma?), I decided to make my own.

And then I had another brainwave, and self-absorbedly wondered if maybe I should start a little custom biz for parents like me who get sick sometimes. They could tell me all about their illness, how it manifests, what they need to do when they get sick so they can get better, and what they want their baby to know.

While every parent's illness will present differently – so all the books will be personalised and bespoke – I'd bet that last one will be an easy copy-and-paste job across every single book. I'd bet that every parent is going to want their baby to know the same thing: that while a parent might get sick sometimes, their baby is the greatest baby and that never changes – and that getting to be a parent is so extra great that when they do feel sick, they do anything they can to hurry up and get better so they can get back to their favourite job.

Here's a first draft. (Please remember I am not a children's book author – I'm barely any kind of author. This is my first book and both this and that are likely crap).

Mummy's Next Door Resting Because She Loves You
by Sinead Corcoran Dye

This is Frank! He has diabetes, which means he needs medicine to make his pancreas work properly so he can be well – and be the best daddy he can be. 👨 💼

This is Morgan! She needs a pacemaker to make her heart work better so she can feel even better and be the best mummy she can be. 👩 🔧

This is Sam! He has hearing aids to make sounds louder for him so he can listen – and be the best daddy he can be. 👨 ✈️

And this is Mum! She takes medicine to make her brain work properly so she can be well – and be the best mum she can be. 👩 ♀️

Sometimes we are born with parts of our bodies not working properly, so we take medicine from when we are just tiny babies. 👼

And sometimes our bodies start out just fine, but then something happens to us later – like a little accident or getting hurt – and we need to start taking the medicine. 💊

Sometimes we take medicine just for a short time, but sometimes we take it for our whole lives, and that's okay! Medicine is so good at making our bodies work properly. 💪

Sometimes if Mums or Dads don't take their medicine or talk about their feelings or take time away to rest, they aren't able to be the best Mums or Dads that they can be.

And we need Mums and Dads to be at their best so they can protect your little brain as it grows into a big brain. 🧠

Because then if you become a Mum or Dad, you will have a big strong brain and can look after all the little brains! 🤗

Mum's medicine helps her brain so much – but sometimes when Big Changes are happening, like a new house or new job, she needs other things to help her too. 🤔

Other things that help Mum's brain are talking to friends, talking to clever doctors, and sometimes going away to rest for a little while. 👨‍👩‍👧‍👦 ⚕️ 😴

But when Mum goes away, she is just in the next room having a little rest and you can come and see her any time you want! 🤗

And when Mum needs to go have a little rest, another mum will always come! 🏃‍♀️

That's one of the very best things about mums – they can be mums to every little person. 🙋‍♀️

Like on the days when you play with Liam and Teddy and Leo and you all have 4 TIMES the mums! 👩🍼👩🍼👩🍼👩🍼❤️

Because your mum and their mums all look after everyone all together so you will have mums FOREVER! 👩👩👩👩❤️

But wait! Here come even more mums! 🏃‍♀️

Here's Hattie and Vanessa and Annabel and Chloe and that's only SOME of your best mums! 👩👩👩👩

And guess what, you will always have so much fun – and fun can even be 4 TIMES the fun! ✨

Because one of these mums is a SUPERMUM! 🦸‍♀️

And two is because this SUPERMUM is your two BEST brothers' mum! 👪💗

So, you can play with them too, and they are always your most favourite fun. 👬⚽

And three is that SuperMum loves to take you for walks to get fluffies and look at all the trees. ☕🌳

And four is she bakes the best CAKES! Yum! 🍰

I know that, usually, going away means someone is saying goodbye. But when Mummy goes away it's so she can actually, very soon, say HELLO I'M BACK!! 🥰

Mummy is just resting her big brain so that she can look after your little brain so that it grows to be SO STRONG. 💪🧠

It is important to take the time to rest so that you can come back and be THE BEST! 🪼

And guess what? Mummy thinks YOU'RE the best and she can't wait to see you soon. 🖤

1 AUGUST 2024 7:46 A.M.

Lara: Happy happy birthday Vivie! Can't wait to celebrate on Sat x

Sinead: Awww thank you. OK unrelated but you know how Stu fucked up my birthday last month and didn't organise a single thing?

Sinead: And then he said he'll make up for it on Vivie's birthday and do a combined birthday treat day for both of us because it's kind of my birthday too because it's the day I gave birth, ya know?

Sinead: Anyway, took too many melatonin pills last night and had nightmares, and one was that for our joint birthday Stu had organised a karate lesson – and was like why are you upset? It was a great deal on GrabOne?

Brooke: My life every day is being asked why I'm upset and I'm like because you're a fucking idiot

Sinead: Also no one is having sex, right? Pls confirm

Lara: Absolutely not. We are exclusively flatmates. I know we need to work on it, but I am eternally tired so maybe tomorrow but probably not.

Brooke: Yup. And I keep being like 'how do I bring this up with him?' And then I think nah CBF, maybe tomorrow. But also, probably not.

Sinead: OK great. Yeah, we're really working on that too – so currently after we get the kids together, we set an hour or two aside for Us Time, which means phones down so we can really connect. And by connect, I mean we snarl at each other for 25–35 mins then retrieve our phones and sit in silence scrolling.

Sinead: And then I'll feel lonely so I'll stretch my foot out towards Stu to try get him to hold hands with my foot and he doesn't – but then at some point he'll accidentally brush past my foot and I'll say DON'T FUCKIN TOUCH ME. So, like, going with the coy, hard-to-get angle you know – supply and demand etc.

Zoe: Yup, I snip at T all day long and then he says in his Italian accent sadly, 'Yes I know I am stupid man,' and then I feel so guilty and apologise and say that I'll try to be nicer to him but then I'm not nicer, because he's a fucking idiot.

Sinead: Don't worry though guys, because I've figured out how we'll get through this and all get our marriages back on track. I've just announced to Stu that 'moving fwd I'm going to operate under the assumption that you were deprived of oxygen at birth. So anything you do – which is always piss-poor – I know is a massive achievement when you've suffered so much brain damage from such a young age.'

Do we want to get divorced or do we just have young children?

AT EXACTLY NINE MONTHS PREGNANT, after a fight with Stu over the fact he still hasn't taught the ten-year-old how to tie his shoelaces, I started looking up studio apartments on TradeMe to move into with our unborn child.

At three months postpartum, after discovering Stu had never actually read the book on emotional labour that I made him buy, I cried and returned to the fantasy apartment search for me and our newborn.

I would go on to hunt for a new rental at least four more times in the first year of Vivie's life when I was sick of Stu's shit. Sick of the crumbs on the bench, sick of how he refuses to download the Solid Starts app (thereby making it my fault alone if we ever poison Vivie with a tomato), sick of him never putting a plastic bag in the bathroom bin and letting Vivie's pissy nappies rot the wicker.

But nothing made me sicker to death of him than his infuriating mumbling that's developed since we welcomed our third child. We assume it's due to tiredness, but at this point I would truly rather he dropped dead onto the ground than suffer through his mumbling a second longer. I spend my days and my nights hissing 'PARDON?!' and trying to Duolingo-style translate his bumbling British – always and forever trailing off into gibberish.

And I am certain beyond a shred of doubt that I am not the only woman having violent thoughts towards my partner – particularly in the first year of babydom.

Take Jessica Grose, a writer for the *New York Times*.

'The lowest point of my marriage was probably when I was excessively pregnant with our second daughter. It was 90 degrees outside every day, and I had blown past my due date with no signs of labor.

'I had trouble falling asleep but had finally drifted off one night when my husband came home from a work event and woke me up. I had a brief and fleeting desire to bludgeon him with a bedside lamp.'[43]

The most relatable content I've come across in a long time.

Relationship researchers John and Julie Gottman found that about two-thirds of couples struggle during the first three years of parenthood, experiencing a noticeable decline in 'relationship satisfaction.'[44]

In the first few months with a new baby, both partners tend to feel unappreciated, intimacy drops off and conflict increases. Although these studies looked only at opposite-sex couples, other research shows that same-sex couples experience similar strains.

'For around thirty years, researchers have studied how having children affects a marriage, and the results are conclusive: the relationship between spouses suffers once kids come along,' said Matthew D. Johnson, Ph.D., author of *Great Myths of Intimate Relationships: Dating, Sex, and Marriage*.[45]

Another thing that drove me wild was that Stu was a fully-functioning, single father of two before I came along. Meaning that, some way or another, even at his house, his children were winter-clothed, had pajamas that fit, had pink shirts for Pink Shirt Day, and had Christmas presents. But as soon as I became the boys' stepmum, suddenly they had no socks unless I sorted them, and it was down to me to organise Easter eggs and Halloween costumes and pocket money and clean duvet covers.

Don't even get me started on the kids' health. I can't even comprehend how the boys survived (at Stu's house; we trust their sensible mother implicitly) with a father who doesn't make a GP appointment unless someone's lost a limb or is bleeding out of their eyes. He once didn't take the little one to the doctor until his legs literally turned purple (it's fine, I promise, because I am the captain now so you don't need to contact any child support services).

When I went to Melbourne for a Taylor Swift concert when Vivie was six months old, I quite seriously told Stu he needed to photograph everything he fed her, along with photos of her holding a thermometer with her current temperature, and that day's newspaper. I was gone for four days.

A 2015 study published in the *Journal of Marriage and Family* showed men did a fairly equal share of the housework—until, that is, they became dads (or in my case, were no longer single dads). Then mums did 13 hours a week more – despite both parents working.[46]

The antenatal class I took never covered postnatal depression – which affects one in five women – or the impact having a baby has on your relationship. Social media is a breeding ground for feeling like you're the only one having a tough time; all you see, for the most part, are idealised highlight reels of smiling parents with giggling babies, and captions about partners being people's 'ride or die' rock. Mums can also be reluctant to open up about the tough times in their relationship with family and friends – particularly girlfriends – fearing it will turn them against their partner.

In terms of the physical labour of running a household (we'll get onto emotional labour soon), Stu and I have adopted a strategy from a 2015 study, published by the Families and Work Institute, that examined 225 same-sex couples: we divide chores according to preference, rather than who 'should' be doing something.[47]

For example, Stu loves cooking (while I loathe it), so he makes us – with the exception of Vivie, as I do enjoy making tiny doll-house food – dinner every night. I, on the other hand, love booking appointments and doing email admin, so I take care of all the organisation for the family. Stu pays all the bills, while I am addicted to shopping and so enjoy making sure everyone has clothes to wear (yes, I know I complained about this earlier). When Vivie is having a screeching meltdown, Stu always takes her away from me as I'm so noise-sensitive that her crying makes me feel like my skin has been set on fire.

While our tasks aren't split 50/50, it does feel relatively equitable. This plan of attack might not work for every couple, but I do rate it – if you can get the perception of fairness right.

Of course, though, there are downsides. If someone is assigned a chore that is equally hated by both parties, well… therein lies the rub. For us, this is the nappy bin, which is Stu's chore – and also writer Jancee Dunn's husband's chore.

'Two months into our daughter's existence, my husband, Tom, and I nearly came to blows over whose turn it was to empty the Diaper Genie, whose plastic entrails had become bloated and coiled like a postprandial Burmese python,' she wrote in her book *How Not to Hate Your Husband After Kids*.

'Normally we're peaceable types, so the volcanic ferocity of our anger surprised us both. I remember glancing down at my hands, clutching the Genie sack, and envisioning them around Tom's neck. When he yelled that he did it "last time," I hollered back that I had carried and delivered the baby "the last time." This was a tired, if effective, retort.'[48]

And while, yes, in theory, male partners have their tasks to complete, I'm also sure I'm not the only mother who often feels that these tasks, in some way or another, end up falling to me to do nonetheless. Because while it's all well and good that Stu has his bits and bobs to do, the household just runs a lot smoother when I do them.

Then there's the emotional labour that commonly falls on mum's shoulders, which includes but is absolutely not limited to:

- Booking all the baby's medical appointments
- Researching what foods to give them and what toys they should play with for their development
- Generally knowing what they need to both survive and thrive

So, yes, Stu does a lot of the physical labour of wrangling her when she's losing it, but he has never once been to Plunket, and could not tell you what developmental 'leap' she's in according to the Wonder Weeks app.

Each task is just a drop in the ocean but together they form a tsunami and it's mums surfing the wave while dads lie on the beach oblivious. Even in couples – like us – who think that they have achieved a relatively equal division of labour, the more hidden forms of care generally end up falling to mum.

Experts say that this invisible, relentless work comes in three overlapping categories.

- Cognitive labour – which is thinking about all the practical elements of household responsibilities, including organising playdates, shopping and planning activities.
- Emotional labour, i.e. maintaining the family's emotions; calming things down if the kids are acting up or worrying about how they are managing at school.
- The mental load is the intersection of the two: preparing, organising and anticipating everything, emotional and practical, that needs to be done to make life flow.

And while we have 'shared' documents on our phones we can each add to, like our grocery and family to-do lists, I'm obviously the one who came up with that idea and worked out how on Earth to add two people to a Notes app doc, and I input all the data and then have to constantly prompt Stu to complete his tasks.

I also came up with the idea (and put into both our calendars) of morning and afternoon 'handover' chats, whereby whoever was 'on shift' gives notes to the other person, and whoever is 'clocking in' asks what the other person needs from them – whether that's tagging into chores or childcare – so the other person can have a break.

I also set up a Sunday night 'week ahead' planning session for the two of us, after becoming sad and resentful that Stu would revolve his work around ensuring he could be at every football game or karate lesson for the boys, while I'd have to do every doctor's appointment or swimming lesson with Vivie. At these planning sessions, we can map out which kid has what on that week, and make sure Stu is present at a fair number of things for each child.

So, I am a stay-at-home mum, a working mum, a housekeeper, a personal assistant to my husband, and a project manager for a team of five – with three of those team members being small children who contribute virtually nothing to our company output. And as I've recently explained to Stu, our house is my office – meaning that if I come downstairs in the morning to a bombsite, it's not just my home that's chaos and anxiety-inducing, it's my workspace that's a mess, too. Do husbands get how utterly unfair and horrible a start to their working day it would be if they turned up to the office and someone had spread junk and toast crumbs across their desk that they had to clean up before they could actually get into their work?

In 2019 Allison Daminger, a doctoral candidate in sociology and social policy at Harvard University, identified four clear stages of mental work related to household responsibilities, and her research found that mothers do a staggering amount more of it across all four stages.[49] These stages include not just identifying what each member of the family needs right this second, but also what they'll likely want and need tomorrow, the next day, for Christmas and for their golden wedding anniversary as well. And the other stages encompass – after identifying these future wants and needs – exhaustively analysing all available options and choosing the best one, i.e. for when the time comes, the most perfectly 'them' wood-stain hue for their casket, à la *Say Yes to the Dress*.

Case in point: while Stu is usually the one to drop Vivie off and pick her up from daycare because it's on his way to work, I'm the one that did all the research on finding a daycare; filled out the applications; managed all the comms with the teacher; created a PDF of her allergies, sleep schedule and emergency contacts; and pack her lunch and her bag every day with the trillion things she needs to take.

Daminger's study also found that married couples didn't argue too much about the household labour split (which would have been a different story if me and Stu were part of the study) in part because women were 'temperamentally interested in being organised' – that they were simply good at planning ahead.[50]

Another case in point: every year, Stu leaves it until two days before his sons' birthdays to order their presents. From the United States. And is then dumbfounded when they don't arrive within twenty-four hours in time for the party. In contrast, I ordered our Christmas tree online the day after I gave birth (when I was still hooked up to a morphine drip) – in August!

The thing is, I don't buy the theory that women are 'just better at that stuff' (planning, organising or multitasking) – I think it's that, even from a young age, we are just expected to do it and so eventually we become better at it.

One analysis, for example, found that boys aged fifteen to nineteen do about half an hour of housework a day, and girls about forty-five minutes. Although girls spend a little less time on chores than they did a decade ago, the time that boys spend hasn't significantly changed.[51]

And as the parents of two boys and a little girl, I'm constantly bleating on at Stu that we need to set an example for them – that Vivie isn't going to be trailing around after them with a little brush and shovel, sweeping up their crumbs.

I don't have the luxury of being a full-time stay-at-home mum (as much as I fantasise about being a tranquilised-on-clonazepam, martini-in-hand housewife). Like most mums in this economy, I must have a job too, and I also have this book I've spent a year writing. So why does everything at home fall to me by default?

My friend Hannah often tells me I'm doing a good job at raising boys who will be self-sufficient enough that women will want to date them. Even when Vivie was a newborn and I had a raw C-section wound, I couldn't stop tidying and cleaning whenever I had a spare minute. While these things calm my anxiety, I also did it because I'm so houseproud and I didn't want visitors coming over and thinking I didn't have my shit together.

In our house, I make sure we have enough nappies in the nappy caddy, play mind-numbingly boring blocks with Vivie, take her to boring-as-batshit ball pits and heartbreaking vaccinations where she bawls in pain. By the time Stu trundles in from work, I'm exhausted and utterly 'over' the baby, so his 'shift' is getting to feed her dinner while she's all happy and cutesy, and showering with her while she cuddles into his neck.

And obviously no one enjoys the nagging.

When I come downstairs in the morning to 'clock in for my shift' and Stu's left the 'workstation' in chaotic disarray with dirty dishes everywhere, baby covered in food sitting in a wet nappy and boys watching football on TV when they haven't fed the cat yet and he's sprinting around screaming, no one's in for a good time. He expects a 'job well done, thanks for managing the kids,' but I'm furious because he's already given me ten chores to jump into when the day has barely begun and it's not even my mess. So Stu feels attacked and I feel like an utter bitch in the process. Good morning!

One Swedish study showed that when women eventually clocked that 'hang on, what the fuck' (re: they're doing absolutely everything around the house), it led to marriage problems and increased the likelihood of a split. And when they deigned to ask for help from their partners (who are grown adults who also reside in said homes), it's dubbed nagging.

'And then that wears on relationships,' says sociologist Daniel Carlson of the University of Utah, and yeah, no shit Daniel, thanks. He also made the groundbreaking discovery that this unequal distribution of caring responsibilities can lead to less sex.[52] I assume he means with each other, because when I once found a lasagne in the oven which had been forgotten about nine days prior, I immediately began planning my future escapades as a single woman.

And in this economy, not all mums can afford to take a year – or longer – of maternity leave, and even fewer can afford to be a stay-at-home mum until their child starts school (if that's something they want).

So, while Stu constantly encouraged me to spend the first few months of Vivie's life resting on the couch, watching TV with her contact napping on my chest, I felt like I had two husbands. That one, and the one who was constantly and openly fretting about our finances, gently asking me if I had any freelance work enquiries this week.

The work pressure piled up, the emotional labour kept piling up, and the laundry kept piling up – all while I had a baby to wrangle, day in and day out. I resented Stu, I resented that I had to work, and I resented that we couldn't afford a full-time cleaner and nanny, so I had to do it all. I just wanted that first husband, who in my fantasy brought home a whopping salary so that all I had to do was take the baby on leisurely walks to the coffee shop and watch endless series of *Keeping Up with the Kardashians*.

As I'm sure you've gathered by now, this first year of having a baby – on top of the two children we already have – has taken an immense toll on our marriage, like it does for many couples.

So, in an attempt to not just be comrade soldiers in the war that is raising children and instead (or also) be a couple, we recently started making date nights a priority. While it doesn't happen every month – because, well, life – we aim to have two 'indoor' dates (once the kids are in bed) and two 'outdoor' dates each month. The outdoor dates are things like going to the movies, or something that requires us to get a babysitter.

We each take turns planning one 'indoor' date that can't just be getting drunk on the couch in front of Netflix – it has to be something creative with effort put in. For example, I did one once where I bought huge canvases and oil pastels and, over a bottle of wine and a cheese platter, we each drew portraits of each other – which turned out ghastly, but also perfect.

And I've already mentioned the Miss Marple incident.

We did nail four dates for the first month because we got on a roll, but it has since petered out because who actually has the energy, and childcare? Who can afford to go out to dinner, pay for Ubers, then pay $100 on top of that for the babysitter? And even if you rely on family members, there's the guilt around 'hey we don't actually have the bandwidth to have you over to wine, dine and small talk because we're exhausted and simply can't be bothered hosting, but would you mind looking after our kids for an evening for free so we can go hang out just us two without you?'

And then there's the whole thing of whether you even want to be near them when date night comes around. If your partner isn't pulling their weight around the house or with the emotional labour of sustaining the relationship and you've been snipping at each other for weeks on end, sitting across from each other at an Asian fusion restaurant isn't exactly going to wave a magic wand over your rage and resentment. You'll most likely sit in near-silence, sending texts to the babysitter checking in on the kids, drinking too much because it's your one night out and you're attempting to be relaxed enough to enjoy your partner's company (and try to forget you lowkey loathe them), only to come home and be – pardon my French – too full to fuck, wake up the next morning hungover and pissed off because you've come downstairs to toast crumbs and filthy children again – and paid almost $400 for the pleasure.

And even when you aren't too full – even if you haven't eaten a crumb – who, may I ask, is actually having sex?

For us, it's similar to our date nights – we can sometimes get on a roll and have sex a few times over the course of a few weeks. Then we'll go months without even a whiff of it in the air, even though we know it's like the gym – you never regret a workout, etc., and if you can find the strength to get up and go, you'll always feel better afterwards. But it's the getting up and going part that bothers me – why would you, when you can lie on the couch and go nowhere?

Last year I interviewed a bunch of new mums on what their sex lives are like now, post having a baby. Their stories were all different, but also all the same.

They all struggled with pain during sex, especially if they'd had a vaginal birth, and they all struggled with their body image: saggy boobs that they didn't want touched anyway because they were still leaking milk – which reminded them they were a mother during an act they really didn't want to associate with being someone's mum. They all had softer, wobbly stomachs which they were self-conscious about, even though their partners had told them they were still beautiful.

And these mums all found it near-impossible to get out of their heads during sex, with a constant merry-go-round of admin spiralling in their heads: Where is that misplaced Plunket book? Did I order my kid's school calendar art? Oh God, I forgot to hang out the wet washing and now it's rotting in the machine.

Plus, after you have a baby, your body feels intrinsically intertwined with that child and with being someone's mum, and it's difficult to rewire your brain to separate the two – a mother and a hot woman who wants to have sex and who someone wants to have sex with.

'My sex drive has kind of plateaued now, to the point I'm consuming all these articles about perimenopause and stuff. I'm like, "why am I so disinterested in it?" But I think it's partly because it became so associated with producing a baby,' one mum who had gone through IVF to have her child told me. 'Sex went from being sexy to making a baby, and it's hard to reverse that. Because making the baby then comes with carrying the baby, birthing the baby and potentially feeding the baby. [Each of] those stages rewired what those parts of my body did for me. So, it became like, "no, no, my vagina, that's where I gave birth, I don't want you down there".

'Before having a baby, I was a real breast person. Afterwards, I didn't want my husband near them. I breastfed for 15 months – those are not pleasure centres [anymore]. I haven't been able to rewire those nerves, I guess. And I feel for my husband – because it's hard to explain and it feels so unfair – but when he initiates sex, I just have these flashbacks of me and my daughter in the dark of the night and feeding her and desperately trying to get her to sleep.'

Another mum explained that her husband not carrying what she believed was an equal share of the load impacted her desire to have sex with him.

'I wish more husbands understood the whole idea of foreplay happening twenty-four hours beforehand. I wish more people could understand the science of what a woman is battling within her own body to try to make it happen. And the feeling of being unsexy and all of that – it is a two-person job to make it happen. And, for me, there is nothing more unattractive than a man that's just, like, slobbing around, not doing anything around the house.'

Advice from many sexperts encourages couples – particularly parents – to schedule sex. But I'm sure you can understand that, as the project manager of our house, family and entire life, who struggles to get my husband to bring the bins in, the idea that I schedule a block in our shared calendar to bring *my* bins in is utterly vagina drying.

So, I've told Stu that he needs to secretly schedule sex in his own brain calendar, so that it's a surprise to me, but this is a man I need to send an @Stu notification to thrice a day to remind him to make a GP appointment for his purple-legged son. So, the sex is obviously not happening.

A while ago I suggested to Stu that perhaps we should see a sex therapist, and he gently replied that no one with a small baby – along with two slightly less small children – is having sex, and perhaps we give it until she's one to see if things pick back up naturally.

I am the toast crumbs, drying out by the day.

I am the empty bins no one is bringing in.

But I am holding on to the idea that none of you are having sex either. This is what helps me sleep at night, in my pajamas no one is taking off (except for me when I am drenched in postpartum sweat – when does that end, please? My child is nearly one and I am never not soaked everywhere on my body, except where we'd all like to be. Sorry, that was quite gross.)

If things don't pick up, I may end up getting that studio apartment off TradeMe and having shared custody of my daughter and I will relish the fact my home will be spotless and free of children half the week. And those few days will also hopefully be filled with sex with many people and in the morning I will make them take the nappy-bin snake on their way out.

INSTAGRAM

MAY 19, 8:47 P.M.

You replied to their story

Ahhh I didn't know we were going out! Gimme ten, are you at Liv's?

Seen

MAY 19, 9:16 P.M.

You replied to their story

Hello hello beep beep where are we heading

Seen

MAY 19, 9:43 P.M.

You replied to their story

Are you still at Hoppers? Lemme know, Stu says he can drop me

Seen

When the weather turned

I DON'T KNOW WHY THIS CHAPTER has been the hardest of all of them to write. I've written about my postnatal depression and having intrusive thoughts of harming my baby and I haven't found it difficult or triggering at all. But this one I've put off until the last minute.

I've written and rewritten it so many times, torn over whether or not to write the ins and the outs of my friendships that slipped away when I got pregnant, and later had Vivie – but I've decided I won't share the stories because it feels unfair when I only have my side to tell.

But what I will say is I think maybe the friendships I lost weren't because I had a baby, I think maybe it's because the foundation of the friendships – based on drinking together and sharing funny TikToks – wasn't strong enough to withstand the storms of my life. In five years, I went from being a sparkly media star and good-time gal, to a very mentally unwell and later physically unwell girl in my pregnancy, then a more mentally unwell mum postpartum.

So, when I started being left out of nights out because I was pregnant – and I'd be on the couch in tears watching my friends having fun without me – I knew that was the beginning of the end.

On reading articles for this chapter, I found an eerily similar experience to mine by Chloe Lovell for *Cosmopolitan* magazine.

'As I scrolled through my feed, stomach churning with the nausea I'd become increasingly accustomed to over the past 14 weeks, I did a double take,' she wrote.

'There, made up in pixels on the screen, was a photo of my six best friends. They were smiling, rosy cheeks pressed up against one another as they merrily sipped cocktails. Sitting at home in my old, dotted pajamas, soft and comforting as a hug, I felt a stab of jealousy. Why hadn't I been invited?

'"We didn't go *out* out," Laura reassured me down the phone the next day. "I just had a few people round, and I know you've not been feeling well lately, so I didn't think you'd want to come."'[53]

But hiding behind the (twelve) copies of that book about the rabbit called *Guess How Much I Love You* that you will receive at your baby shower is often grief, and jealousy. 'Friendships do change once one person has a child,' Anna Mathur, psychotherapist and author of *Raising a Happier Mother*, says. 'It switches the dynamics.'

She rationalises that there can be a sense that you've lost that person to motherhood.

'There can be jealousy and envy on both sides,' she explains, and a social expectation to hide these feelings can often result in miscommunication, or even assumptions. 'We often tell ourselves stories in friendships about what the other person is thinking or feeling.'[54]

According to a study of 2,000 people conducted by UK charity Action for Children a few years ago, over 68 per cent of parents feel 'cut off' from friends after the arrival of a baby.[55]

And I've read plenty of think-pieces where child-free women have ditched friendships with mums and their flaky, unpredictable schedules, or about how mums no longer have the time to constantly maintain group chats or the energy to go on nights out.

And I'm sure that's the case for lots of friendships – but that wasn't the case for me. Even in my craziest, most sleep-deprived newborn days, I was always up for a night out (I'm a party animal) and always replied to messages instantly – a child in one hand and my phone permanently glued to the other. So maybe it wasn't that I was simply no longer available, maybe it was that I was available but too much had changed. Life had gotten so much harder; I had gotten sicker in every way and now a baby was here.

Sometimes these friendships disintegrate because it's too painful to continue them if one person has a new baby and the other desperately longs for one – approximately one in four New Zealanders experience infertility and one in eight require some form of medical assistance to achieve a pregnancy.[56]

While I'll never know for sure if that was the reason why, one close friend who I've known for a decade has drifted away from me since I had Vivie. In the months after I had her, I tried to arrange brunches and dinners with this friend – but there was always a reason she couldn't come to them, and she didn't attend my baby shower either.

Trish Elliott, a woman in the United States who desperately yearns to become a mother, explained to *Today* why it's too hard to stay friends with people – particularly mums who work full-time – who have children when she doesn't.

'I didn't want to go out with my friends anymore. I was having lots of headaches and became very depressed,' she said. 'I thought my marriage was going to end because all we did was argue. Everything seemed to revolve around having a baby. More friends and family became pregnant and baby shower invitations came in the mail. I couldn't go to them. I tried once, but I sat in the parking lot in tears and had to leave. I just didn't understand.'[57]

I desperately miss that close friend, but I understand and respect her decision to look after herself and would never want me or my daughter's presence to cause her pain.

Mathur also says that at times, to protect yourself and the

friend from further hurt, it can be best to try and accept that some relationships can't withstand such a monumental life change.

'Perhaps the linchpin has been nights out, or lunches at work and you start to realise that these friendships were built on prominent features that are no longer relevant to your life anymore,' she says.[58]

And it's not just mums whose social circles shrink after their baby arrives. According to a recent survey, a growing number of men are losing close friends within the first year of having a child. In 2019, the Movember Foundation commissioned research of 4,000 men across Canada, the UK, USA and Australia that investigated their social connections, specifically emphasising parenthood and the impact of becoming a father.

The report found that 20 per cent of fathers said the number of close friends they had decreased in the twelve months since becoming a father. Furthermore, 33 per cent of men with no good friends said their stress levels increased a lot compared with 23 per cent of those with at least one close friend.[59]

There's that old overused saying that 'people come into your life for a reason, a season, or a lifetime' and I think this is true. Then there's that unequivocally-not-used-enough saying 'You look like a boozer and a slob. Have you ever even had sex? Sometimes you are mistaken for a bloke, aren't you?' and not a truer word has ever been spoken.

The concept of a capsule wardrobe, a curated collection of versatile, timeless essentials was originally coined by London boutique owner Susie Faux in the 70s. But Susie was an absolute nobody so no one gave a fuck and just went about their lives. That was, until 2001 when two British fashion advisors emerged from the unholy depths of hell to launch a BBC makeover series with a firm philosophy that one must forgo fleeting trends and seasonal shifts – and instead invest in a curated collection of staples. Those year-round, year-in and year-out investment pieces that you love and always make you feel good – the ones you'll reach for time and time again.

Just like all the best things, these capsule pieces are actually the most valuable things in your wardrobe. Kind of like those two-dollar-shop plastic ponchos that are actually the most valuable thing on Earth when it starts pissing down on the Fyre Festival that is the human existence. And when life does start getting a bit too Fyre Festival-y, what you really need is a plastic poncho of a friend.

Because life is not fair, so what good is a fair-weather friend when dark clouds start to roll in? From here on out you must only have friends that are waterproof and wind-resistant.

I didn't know that back then. But I know that now. And I still have my Now & Thens.

Twenty years ago, a little girl group of me and my three best friends were just like the girls in the movie: Roberta, Teeny, Samantha and Chrissy. Except instead of playing in a treehouse and telling our parents we were having a sleepover when we were actually doing seances in cemeteries (WOAH CALM DOWN YOU CRAZY CATS!), we would tell our parents we were having a sleepover and then go get blackout drunk in the park across the road from school.

Other nights we would don our Supré singlets that we had personalised by graffitiing our 'tagger' names in neon across the chest – despite never having tagged anything in our lives. (My tagger name was '$inBaddd' which at the time I coined to convey that I was both sinful and a 'baddie', and only now at the time of writing this I realise people most likely assumed it was a nod to the cartoon Arabian sailor man who spent his life sailing the seven seas.)

Pimped-out in our singlets, denim cut-offs and approximately eleven decorative belts that served nary a function, we would tootle off to renowned underage Christian club, Yellow Brick Road, where we would down party pills and dance seductively to entice our acne-riddled male counterparts. (And by seductively, I mean thanks to the 'lucky dip' medley of pills, we would spend the entire evening with our eyes closed, slumped against a wall.)

And as *Your Love Never Fails* by Neon Feather & NEON Worship and *Step into the Fight (Gregatron Remix)* reverberated through the church, and the power of *Goodness of God (Remix)* by Gui Brazil compelled us, only our heads rhythmically bobbed up and down to the music, like nodding dogs on a dashboard.

Twenty years later, when I was pregnant and the head bobbing days were a distant memory, I became part of another 'for better or for worse' foursome - and all we had in common was our postcode and our due date. If I could recommend anything to a pregnant person, it would be laxatives, but it would also be to do an antenatal class. I have only survived the last year because of the women I met – women who I drink with, cry with and text at 2 a.m. saying, 'Hey I'm not loving this,' and they reply saying 'Don't worry, me neither.' A group of women who don't have to pretend they're 'soaking up every moment,' because not every moment is good – so many are shit – but they're a lot less shit when you have friends in it with you too.

Friends who say they're struggling too, and remind you that you're not alone.

I haven't been alone for a long time because I have really good staples.

Kate, Shannan, Diana, my mums' group.

My best friend Hannah - who is Vivie's godmother and is the world's worst godmother. In the two years since she was appointed this holy and prestigious honour, she has never babysat Vivie once. I'm often not even halfway through an utterly unrelated sentence about something like yoghurt - not even in a question format - when she panics and screams 'I'm actually at capacity right now and I'm really not interested in looking after someone else's child thanks!?!' She also turned up to her god-daughter's first birthday party three hours late, repulsively hungover in a tracksuit with the hood up and sunglasses on. She brought no gift. She also smelled and looked like one of the three blind mice.

Hannah is the world's best godmother. Because Stu is my person but if there was ever no Stu, I would still be fine because there is never no Hannah, keeping me tethered to the world. So, I never float away, because Hannah is always with me. She is the world's best godmother because she keeps me alive so I won't be dead. Ergo, there will never come a time where Vivie will have to utilise her pitiful godmother services and live with her = Vivie will continue to live.

Shortly after my mum died, I lost touch with my aforementioned Now & Then friends. Because I tried to run. As far away from that house and that life as I could. Those friends were all about me and them, and me and them and her. And there was no me anymore without her, and so many pages in the book of my life about them and her – so I had to rip all those pages out.

I made new friends who hadn't read the book before.

I once had a professional photoshoot done for something I was working on at the time, and the photo editor, who I can only assume was a former *What Not To Wear* staffer, must have deemed me so utterly grotesque that 'less is more' was simply not an option when it came to my touch-ups. And upon seeing the truly violently photoshopped published images, my friend Annabelle said I looked so fucked up 'like I was about to blast off into space.'

She has also said this about every photo I've posted on Instagram since.

A few months ago, we all went out for dinner and I made a wry gag about 'remember that time I actually did blast the fuck off and didn't even say bye hahaha.'

And she said 'No, you didn't that time. You just got lost for a little bit. But it's OK because we found you.'

The phrase 'less is more' in terms of choosing quality over quantity in all areas of life is often attributed to Ludwig Mies van der Rohe, a renowned German-American architect. But there's an even more poignant phrase that has always stuck with me – reminding me why I have long retired my Nights Out dresses in favour of the cosy and comfortable – pieces built to last, and get even better with time:

'That dress is like a bad relationship: It makes you look bloated, and it doesn't even have the decency to support you. And also, that's not a dress, that's a sofa with a zip.' Trinny Woodall.

30 MAY 2024, 9:16 P.M.

Sinead: Hey Annie, it was so nice chatting again on Zoom last night and once again we're so, so grateful you're doing this for us. So, we met with our fertility clinic today and they can do our group appointment in two weeks, then we'll move onto our individual counselling sessions – then a joint one all together. After that me and Stu will put our surrogacy application in through both the ethics committee and Oranga Tamariki – but we don't anticipate any hold up there. And they've confirmed they can courier the embryos to your clinic in Wellington, and once the baby is born, we'll go through the adoption process. Gah it's a lot I know, and again – we can't thank you enough x

Seen

15 JUNE 2024, 6:34 P.M.

Stuart: Hey Annie, just wanted to check in

Seen

You've got a match!

I HADN'T EVEN HAD VIVIE when I raised the idea with Stu of using a surrogate to carry our next child.

As soon as Vivie was born in August, I was already researching the process and the legalities behind it. I learned that it would be an incredibly difficult and lengthy process with tons of hoops to jump through – and that's if we could even find someone.

I read that the process could take a couple of years, if not more, so made Stu promise that we could get started the following January. But January came and went, as Stu wasn't emotionally ready to even contemplate having a fourth child – particularly after the pregnancy and postpartum nightmare I'd had. That had been traumatic for him, too.

As I mentioned previously, Stu is an incredibly private person and confided in me that he had a huge wall up regarding the idea of a stranger carrying his child – he said he couldn't fathom why on Earth someone would do such a thing altruistically with no payment.

I explained that, unlike him (someone who would never give

spare change to a homeless person on the street), many people get a lot out of helping others – whether that's through buying a pin on Daffodil Day, volunteering at a shelter, or maybe even carrying a child. But he still had reservations and said he was suspicious of anyone who would do such a thing.

I became increasingly frustrated that he was dragging his heels on getting started.

'You promised me we could have another baby,' I'd yell, and he'd reply that he didn't remember that being the agreement. Every night after the kids were in bed we'd have heated whisper-arguments, never able to agree on what we'd agreed years prior.

While I'd love nothing more than for someone else to carry my baby, because I utterly loathed being pregnant, I did have secret fears too. Like, what if something went wrong or she miscarried – would I blame her? And, what if we went through the lengthy and expensive counselling process only for her to pull out at the last minute? Or, my worst fear of all, what if she decided to keep the baby, and we wouldn't be able to do a thing about it because legally it would be her child until we adopted?

My therapist suggested that, together, Stu and I should write out a 'pros, cons and fears' list regarding having another baby, which Stu eventually agreed to. But after I added a fourth column – 'solutions' – he snapped at me that, 'If you're going to try to "solve" every one of my cons with a solution then you're basically saying the decision is made.' The exercise ended in another fight, too.

But Stu would later go on to see a therapist himself, to talk about the trauma he still held around the journey to get Vivie, his concerns about my mental health and the impact that two young children would have on that, fears of aging without having freedom for another two decades, and his pressing concerns about the state of our finances. On arriving home from a session, he said the therapist had been helpful and that he felt ready to have another baby. I kissed him, cried and said thank you.

That afternoon I joined Love Makes a Family, a matchmaking

organisation founded by a gay couple after successfully welcoming two children via egg donation and surrogates. The agency pairs up hopeful families with donors who offer up their eggs, sperm or wombs.

I scoured the available surrogates like they were potential Tinder matches, swiping left on anyone who looked a bit 'dodgy' or had a poorly written profile. I'd also only swipe right on women who lived in Auckland, as the idea of our baby being in another city freaked me out, and we wouldn't be able to afford to fly back and forth anyway.

I'd quickly discover that choosing a surrogate is not like choosing a lonely, 'in desperate need of a home' cat from the SPCA – the surrogates are the ones who choose, not the families. And the number of families seeking donors outweighs the number of donors about a million to one, and there's not enough to go around.

After receiving no replies from the nice, wholesome-looking Auckland-based surrogates, I wrote to the 'dodgy' ones too, telling myself that just because someone looks a bit sketchy and has terrible tattoos, that doesn't make them a bad person or baby carrier.

I still got no replies.

So, I spent hours emailing every single surrogate on the website, even ones that lived so far away from Auckland that it may as well have been Timbuktu.

Weeks went by and, still, nothing. I started to panic.

I forced Stu into letting us have professional photos taken of us by a photographer friend at his work, persuading him that 'marketing was everything' when it came to attracting 'a good buyer'. Much to his reluctance, he let me share the photos on Instagram as an ad, with a caption explaining our story and our desperate need for a surrogate. Thanks to the incredible generosity of my social media community, the post was shared far and wide – reaching over 40,000 people.

We had a handful of women get in touch saying they would be happy to do it for us, but for one reason or another they all changed their minds. Which we understood; it's a huge decision and a huge deal to sacrifice nine months of your life and put your body on the line for two strangers and no personal gain. But after taking two of these women out for brunch and paying for their meals, only to have them pull out, we were disheartened.

There are many reasons people might need a surrogate. Mine, as you know by now, is the risk to me and to any baby I might carry. Kiwi TV presenter Toni Street turned to surrogacy as she suffers from a rare autoimmune disease that inflames blood vessels, which meant she couldn't carry the baby herself.[60] Same-sex male couples need a surrogate if they are to have a baby. And globally, infertility is on the rise which is fuelling an increase in surrogacy.[61]

A Law Commission report in 2022 concluded 'a pressing need for reform'. It made a series of recommendations which – while maintaining the ban on commercial surrogacy – would act to 'safeguard the rights and interests of surrogate-born children, surrogates and intended parents'.

'The [current] law fails to meet the needs and reasonable expectations of New Zealanders in many respects.'[62]

Celebrities like Chrissy Teigen, Elizabeth Banks, Anderson Cooper and Jamie Chung have been open about their experiences with surrogacy and largely praised the process despite ethical concerns raised by some advocates, who say paying a woman to have a child opens her up to exploitation by wealthier and more powerful intended parents.

While attitudes towards surrogacy are changing, it remains a minefield of complex legal, ethical, cultural and medical issues. And lawmakers and politicians appear to prefer to dodge the laws that govern surrogacy in New Zealand – they haven't been updated for almost seventy years.

I recently connected with Mark Edwards and Christian Newman, the founders of the agency I mentioned, Love Makes a Family. The couple met at Wellington's 'one and only gay bar,' and a few years later they began investigating how to make their dreams of having a family a reality. But they quickly realised it wasn't going to be easy, or cheap. As a gay, male couple, their only options were adopting or surrogacy. After three years of trying to start their family and spending more than $50,000, the couple welcomed their first child, a son called Frankie, born via surrogacy in 2018. But despite Frankie being their biological son, they then had to enter into a lengthy and expensive legal battle to adopt him.

'Bringing a child into the world should be a really joyful and exciting and fun experience,' says Newman. 'It's exhausting and tiring enough having a newborn, so to have to go and deal with lawyers and go through an adoption process just because we're a same-sex couple is just so unfair.'

Newman has been battling to change the system so that no other couple has to face the emotional and financial toll that he and his husband did. 'The cost is prohibitive for a lot of intending parents, some people can't even afford to go through this whole process to have a child,' he says.

There are myriad barriers to the surrogacy process:

- There's no single source of authoritative information in New Zealand – instead a hotchpotch of amateur support services.
- Funding for fertility technologies hasn't increased since 2006, which restricts the number of patients fertility specialists can take on.
- There are inconsistencies in who can access what funding is available.
- There's no register for surrogacy, so matching intended parents with potential surrogates is all but impossible.
- There's a limited number of lawyers with experience in surrogacy issues.

The list goes on.

However, the biggest problem for Newman – and many others who have been through the process – is adopting the new baby.

Overseen by Oranga Tamariki (OT) through the Family Court, the process takes months, costs tens of thousands of dollars, and involves OT check-ins, house visits and a written report supplied to the court before approval to adopt is given.

Newman, who went through it twice to have their second child, Lulu, in 2021, described it as incredibly invasive. 'They come into your house a number of times. They ask questions that are really invasive, around your financial security, around your religion, your dogs, your dog's breed, your parents' relationships, any physical [or] sexual abuse in your family, verbal abuse, what your parents were like, what schools you went to, what your relationships with your family and your brothers and sisters are like.

'It feels like it's an interrogation. And in essence, the thing that underpins it all is they're trying to ascertain whether or not we would be proper and fit parents. And again, it's really unfair. It's not something that everyone else must deal with. It's only people that are going through this reproductive process in order to have kids. They've already struggled for years to have kids. It's a costly and expensive process. And then you've got these people invading your home and you have to be on your best behaviour and all the rest of it to get a tick of approval for you to have children.'

The idea that we, a loving family in an expensive suburb with three healthy, cared-for and thriving children, need to be assessed by an organisation responsible for children in harm feels horrific, and unfair.

We also really want our children to be as close in age as possible, and as Stu approaches fifty, the clock ticks. If we can't find a woman willing to carry for us in the next few months, devastatingly I may have no other choice but to get pregnant again – which fills me with terror, and heartbreak for my daughter. I can't bear the idea of her having a mum who can't get out of bed, who can't chase her around the playground or lift her up anymore.

I'm writing this chapter in June 2024, and by the time you read this I may be pregnant. I may be midway through a book tour, press events and signings, while running outside to vomit in alleyways, with skin the colour of cement, dead eyes I can barely keep open and a body skinnier than before I was carrying a baby. And that fills me with terror.

And we are just one of the many families desperate for the generosity of strangers.

12 JULY 2021, 7:40 A.M.

Sinead: How's the game going?

Stuart: 1-1 and just started extra time. Hey did you sleep OK? I woke a lot and you were awake every time?

Sinead: yea I not feeling ver well

Stuart: Oh no! Have you tried eating something? Maybe low blood sugar?

Sinead: Oh yeah, I forgot the doctor said I shouldn't just have smoothies.

Stuart: Yup that will be it.

Sinead: OK all good love you.

Stuart: Love you too.

9:32 A.M.

Sinead: Hey sorry to be annoying I know this is worst time for this to hap but do you think you coming home soon? I feels worse now. I've been vomiting all morning and I'm so hot but then I get so cold

Stuart: Oh no! We will get you to the doctor on Monday x

Sinead: No, I need to see someone today

Stuart: OK we will get you seen today x

Sinead: I'm so sorry this is happening now. It's OK I'm fine, we'll talk after the game x

11:41 A.M.

Sinead: Will you be home soon?

Stuart: Will just finish this beer then come home x

Sinead: Actually, no you should stay, don't want you to come home

Stuart: Why? Cause I'll drunkenly hug you and you'll be irritated by my drunkenness hehe

Sinead: Stu I'm not normal that's what I'm trying to say

Sinead: Something is really wrong

Sinead: I'm so sorry this is happening at the worst time but I need you to come home I'm panicking

Stuart: Omfg I'm so sorry I didn't realise it was this bad I'm so sorry, I'm trying to find an Uber now

12:45 P.M.

Sinead: Are you coming

Sinead: Where are you

Sinead: Please please come home

Living the dream

THE WEEK BEFORE MY TWENTY-NINTH BIRTHDAY, my brain snapped and I thought that jumping off my balcony was the only way I could escape from it. I can now see that it had been breaking down for a while.[63]

Every time I got a slight twinge or noticed a tiny irregularity in my body, I would be googling cancer symptoms. I scoured WebMD at least three times a day. I made doctors' appointments every other week; there was never anything wrong with me but, despite their ever-patient reassurance, I never believed them.

I know now that my mum's death from breast cancer was the catalyst for this – but at the time I was convinced I was undiagnosed with a tumour, slowly killing me, that no doctor had spotted. In reality, it was a poison in my brain.

I've always been prone to bouts of anxiety, but in the months leading up to my birthday my worrying snuck out of control. I say snuck, because I didn't spot it at the time. Neither did Stu. I think when you're so familiar with your own anxious brain – or your partner's mad hypochondria – you don't spot red flags.

At that time, I was under a lot of stress at work and had stopped sleeping. After a recent back injury resulting in a trapped nerve, I had become fixated on the idea that I was going to have to have my leg amputated. I would also ask Stu to examine my body parts under his iPhone torch to check for signs of cancer.

The day my brain snapped I was rabid in my internet search for proof of the fatal disease killing me. After four hours of constant googling, I tried to make myself stop by having a shower. A minute later, I had to get out to fetch my phone so I could google while I showered. That's the last thing I remember before everything changed.

I don't know if it was a slow dimming of the lights in my brain or if they switched off instantly – all I remember is feeling like I'd drunk two bottles of wine all at once.

I got out of the shower, and everything was almost cartoon-like. I was moving in slow motion. I looked at myself in the mirror but I couldn't focus. I was just a shape, no detail.

I knew I had been hot in the shower, but I felt no sensation of heat in my body. I bit down on my hand so hard it bled. Still, nothing.

I knew where I was – I was in the bathroom. But I wasn't really in the bathroom. The bathroom wasn't real.

I came to the conclusion that I must be asleep, and this was a dream. Except a few minutes ago I had been awake. So how had I fallen asleep in the shower? And why wasn't the water waking me up?

All I knew for certain was that something had gone very, very wrong. And I was convinced it was my fault.

Derealisation was first used as a clinical term more than 120 years ago, yet it remains widely misunderstood.

Daphne Simeon, who led a depersonalisation clinic specialising in many different psychotherapy and psychopharmacological treatments, co-wrote a book on the disorder. In the book, titled

Feeling Unreal, she quotes from Joanne, a patient: 'I'd really rather have cancer than this. With a disease that people know, you can get some degree of empathy. But if you try and explain this, people either think you're crazy or completely self-absorbed and neurotic. So, you keep your mouth shut and suffer silently.'[64]

In comedian and actor Bo Burnham's award-winning Netflix special *Inside*, Burnham mentioned the psychological phenomenon of derealisation, sparking a wave of interest in the condition.[65] The show – a mix of music, comedy and powerful introspection – came after the American star's previous revelations of his battles with mental health, depression, anxiety and dissociation.

My psychiatrist, Dr Giselle Rausch, describes derealisation as an experience of feeling detached from your surroundings, in a dreamlike or lifeless state.

'Depersonalisation and derealisation (DPDR or dissociative disorder) commonly coexist with a mood disorder – namely depression, anxiety and post-traumatic stress disorders. Symptoms are often triggered or evoked by stress or fatigue causing significant distress and interference with a person's ability to function.'

Unlike other psychotic disorders, people with DPDR know that their experiences of detachment aren't real – which makes it all the more frightening.

About fifty per cent of the general population have had at least one transient experience of depersonalisation or derealisation in their lifetime. For most people, it's basically like zoning out when you're driving and not remembering the drive home.

However, only about two per cent of people meet the criteria for having DPDR, where episodes can last for hours, days, weeks or even months.

Often, people with DPDR have experienced trauma in their lives, including emotional or physical abuse or neglect in childhood. My understanding of it is people like me develop DPDR in childhood as a protective measure to shut their brain down when what's going on around them is too much to bear.

For me, it manifests as a surreal dream state, like I'm really drunk – except it's not fun at all. It mostly affects my vision. I'm unable to adjust my eyes to look at things in the foreground, and I lose all feeling in my body – I can't feel ice, or boiling water, pain or pleasure. I also have no attachment to my short- or long-term memories; they just feel like episodes of a show I watched a long time ago.

At the peak of my first episode the week before I turned twenty-nine, I became so convinced I was dreaming that I thought I needed to jump off our apartment deck to wake up. It was at that point I called the mental-health crisis team, and their incredible staff spent the next eight hours on the phone with me while I screamed and shook and cried. While for a long time I had felt nothing, it had been a long time now – and now I was also in so much pain. My body had started to seize up from shaking with fear. I was almost immediately diagnosed with DPDR, and I've been an outpatient at the Taylor Centre ever since, while they try to find medication that will keep my episodes at bay. But therein lies the rub – there is no exact treatment for DPDR.

Because it's an extreme version of anxiety and panic, the prevailing school of thought is that the best chance at minimising episodes is through talk therapy, cognitive behavioural therapy, antidepressants and anti-anxiety medications. So, in the year after that first episode, it was trial and error when it came to finding a medication that might help prevent or at least minimise the severity of my flare-ups – and the first medication we tried made me gain thirty kilograms.

I went from a size ten to a size sixteen. None of my clothes fit anymore and I lost all confidence in my appearance. And despite quickly changing to another med, the weight stuck around for years. It's only recently, since going on ADHD medication – which often suppresses appetite – that the weight has fallen off and I look like myself again, with the addition of post-baby stretch marks, looser skin and sad, droopy bags-of-Pitango-soup tits.

I resent my mental illness a lot, particularly as it's likely something that developed due to childhood trauma and situations that were completely out of my control. It feels really shitty that those circumstances have now impacted my quality of life and, in turn, my career.

I used to work in busy newsrooms and on TV sets, but those environments became impossible for me once I started having all-consuming episodes because, when they kick off, I become really sensitive to noise and fluorescent lights. In the years that followed my diagnosis, I tried multiple different jobs across the media industry, and none stuck. The first day at these jobs would always be okay, because I'm good at meeting and greeting new people, but as soon as I got handed a piece of work, the anxiety and the dissociative waves would start rolling in, and my vision would go blurry and distorted. The office would feel like a maze of mirrors. While trapped in an episode, I'd often lose my spatial awareness and end up with scrapes and bruises up my arm from bumping into walls and furniture.

The final nail in the coffin that was my career as I knew it was in the throes of an episode at a new job – I had to feign a cold so I could go home, and crashed my car on the way because I could barely see. That's when I knew it was over. The career I had built over a decade just washed down the drain.

After taking a few months to try and recover my pride, I became a freelance writer, which gave me the freedom to work from home in my quiet, comfortable space, and only work when I wanted to or when I was well enough. At the time we were in a financial position where we could afford for me to stop working when I needed to have a break, and for that I'm really grateful. It terrifies me to think, what if this had happened to me when I was single and flatting with no parents to support me?

When I am having an episode, I cancel plans unless they're with very close friends who understand my illness. Group hangouts and family dinners can be hard for me as it's lots of people talking all at once, which can be too much for my brain, so these days I find it easier to spend time with people one-on-one.

I also don't go anywhere that's overly stimulating, like supermarkets or shopping malls, and I avoid driving as it's terrifying when you can't see properly. I'll also have lots of hot showers to try and reconnect the split wires between my brain and body, and hold Vivie or sit next to Stu as much as possible – he's the human equivalent of a weighted blanket. Having kids in my house also helps, as nothing jerks you back to the present quite like constantly bleating children or a baby spitting into your mouth for a treat.

'The symptoms of depersonalisation and derealisation can be countered with the same treatments used to battle anxiety disorders,' says Giselle.

That means a combination of psychotherapy to manage the underlying causes, and medication to fight the 'underlying neurobiology' – inflammation of the brain due to stress hormones.

Since being diagnosed I've tried multiple types of therapy and countless combinations of medications. And while they do help a bit, I haven't found a cure yet. My best chance at avoiding episodes now is avoiding my triggers, like stress, exhaustion, overwhelm and panic.

Having a mental illness is isolating enough, but having one that no one's heard of is even more so. I initially joined a Facebook group for people with DPDR, and it was great for feeling less alone, but it was also a really scary, sad place. It's full of frightened, sick people and desperate pleas for a cure, and horror stories about those who have been stuck in episodes for years on end.

A couple of years ago I was put on a new medication called Lamotrigine, which helped enormously. While I still had episodes, they were less frequent and less crippling. And then one day, they stopped altogether – the week I got pregnant.

For those nine long months, despite being mentally and

physically annihilated in every which way, I didn't have a single blip of dissociation. My psychiatrist Giselle thinks two things shielded me – and Vivie – from it, right up until she was born.

The first was that the root cause of dissociation is not being present in your body because your brain has been wired to believe it's not a safe place to be, which is why grounding exercises are often recommended to sufferers. Because I was so violently ill in my pregnancy, there was no way I could drift off when I was constantly crippled with migraines, body aches and vomiting, I was forced to be excruciatingly present in my body at all times, whether I liked it or not.

Giselle thinks the other reason was to protect Vivie.

According to scientific research, during pregnancy, some autoimmune issues, like arthritis, can hit pause. This happens because a specific enzyme, pyruvate kinase, goes down, which tones down the immune system's usual intensity.[66]

Sometimes, the immune system can be a bit too keen and accidentally attacks healthy cells. But with less pyruvate kinase flowing, it chills out, allowing the body to focus on growing the baby instead. And researchers are now looking into whether they can mimic this effect to help people with autoimmune diseases feel better, even when they're not pregnant.

I can't find anything online about something similar occurring with women who suffer from dissociative disorders, but I've decided it can. At least it can to me, for her. Because I can count the severe flare-ups I've had since having Vivie on one hand.

After we got through the sleepless newborn period and I was getting eight hours again, and now armed with a toolkit of things I know help me, I'm much better equipped when the episodes do smack me down like a wave. But I think the biggest reason the spells happen so infrequently now is because I'm not frightened of them anymore.

I know when the wave hits, instead of panicking and thrashing around – which, as we know, can cause you to drown – I need to stretch out onto my back, shut my eyes and just let it carry me, doing its thing. I know the more loosey-goosey I can be, the gentler the ride and the sooner I'm back on shore. I know that no matter how frightening waves can be, even tsunamis roll into shore soon enough.

In the years following my diagnosis, I found ways of coping. I initially went absolutely Gwyneth on it, quitting coffee and booze and trying to meditate and journal, but it didn't stick. I'm too tired, and also too bored, and also too addicted to dopamine to cut all those great things and pick up wholesome habits. Because I am a piece of shit!

The only one recommended to me that I still do to this day is TIPP skills – Temperature change, Intense exercise, Paced breathing and Progressive muscle relaxation. These are used to 'connect back with your body and your surroundings,' says my clinical psychologist, Shruti Pathak.

'If you feel your emotions getting out of control or feel yourself dissociating, you can use the TIPP skills to help ground you.'

For example, when I feel like I'm starting to dissociate, I'll usually take a clonazepam then put a bag of frozen peas on my face while I wait for the medication to kick in. I'll then squeeze my hands into fists and breathe in for three seconds and out for seven, then do a few star jumps or run on the spot.

Pathak says these techniques help to lower the intensity of your emotions and bring you back to the present, distract from whatever is triggering you, 'help focus on what is going on inside your body and can bring you outside of the emotions that may lead to dissociation'.

And because fuck never drinking again and fuck journalling (I write all the time? It is my literal job to write words for money? I am obviously not going to write some more for free?) – I have come up with my own tools for my own toolkit.

While these are very specific and bespoke to me and the things that bring me joy and peace, I will include them here. Just in case you'd like some inspo and also some reassurance that your own Tool Things don't have to be yoga and sound baths (I did one once and it sounded like dementors ricocheting through the sky to suck my soul?) – your Tool Things can be whatever wacky shit you like.

My special Tool Things

Hot shower
So hot your skin is worryingly red and borderline blistered when you emerge. Extra good if, while showering, your husband sits on the toilet (like on the lid, not actually using it) to keep you company with chitty chats.

Two dowdy wheat packs
One draped across the front of your neck like a bad scarf, one resting on your tum.

Re-watching *Friends* for one trillionth time
Ep recs include:

- The one where Rachel is dating Ross's girlfriend's dad played by Bruce Willis and Ross hides from him by slithering behind the bed like a shot snake
- The one where Ross accidentally gets multiple spray tans all layered on top of each other
- The one where Ross screams 'Pivot!!' at Chandler while they're moving a couch
- The one where Ross drinks margaritas to cope with Rachel dating Joey and keeps screaming 'I'm FINE!!'
- Basically, any episode with Ross being all of us

Playing Ratchet & Clank on PlayStation
This game was released in 2002 when I was ten, and as an only child this 'anthropomorphic alien creature known as a Lombax'[67] (named Ratchet) and escaped robot (named Clank) were often my

only companions. Sitting alone in my dark, sweltering living room with the curtains closed, saving the galaxy from 7 a.m. to 7 p.m. all weekend long while perched on a chocolate-stained beanbag sipping Vanilla Coke was my ten-year-old self's life purpose, my life's true joy. If I could teleport back to any moment in my life, it would be this, every time. Which is why when I'm sick, I trundle off down to the playroom and climb aboard my 2D rocket ship once more and travel through the cartoon universe, saving it from evil forces – until you kill all the forces then have to reboot the game and do it all again, even though you're a 32-year-old mother and your children are upstairs saying to their dad 'what do you mean Sinead's gaming?'

Let me tell you: it's because when you are zooming across the galaxy fighting crime, flanked by your two best compadres (drawings of a Furry and a very small robot), you are ten again, AKA an age before you were sick.

The makers of Ratchet & Clank have just released a brand-new version of this game, but it's only available on PS5. So, to tide me over until we hopefully come into many riches, I am one of those very sad people who watch people play a game on YouTube, and I wonder if I am just one step away from those other kinds of people who actually use VR porn.

Calling Kate or Hannah (or both)

They are my two best friends and, apart from Stu, the only people I feel okay conversing with when I'm in the throes of an episode – because when I hear myself speaking it sounds like I'm underwater, like the haunting sound of merpeople, and it makes me panic that What if it sounds like that to other people too? But even if I am a merman, Kate and Hannah don't care, they just roll with it.

Eating nostalgic food (must have crunch)

Anything you ate as a child that wasn't your mum's shit dinners. My go-tos are Fairy Bread, syrup on toast or this drink my mum invented (probably not) called Milkypops – some random concoction of honey, cinnamon and milk – and maybe weed?

Stu, bless him, is forever trying to perfect the recipe to make it exactly how my mum's was – minus the maybe weed.

Having my hair brushed

When my mum lost hers, she relished my long hair even more. In the afternoons during my final year of university, I would perch on the end of her hospital bed while she brushed it, making me promise I'd never shave it off for any 'fundraising rubbish'.

And when I had a severe panic attack at my flat one night when she was about to die, one of my flatmates phoned her aunt, whose mum had also died of cancer. She told her aunt it was an emergency, and when the aunt got to our flat, she yanked me outside onto the deck, popped me down on the floor between her knees and brushed my hair, hard. Hard in the Thai massage kind of style, where it hurts but in a good way, so you can really feel it. The aunt must have known that if I could really feel something – anything – I would come back to myself. So now, if in doubt, I brush. Or Stu brushes his little frightened pony.

Temu

If you haven't heard of Temu, I believe you must live in a bunker. But I'm going to tell you anyway, bunker-dweller or not.

The U.S. offshoot of Chinese e-commerce giant Pinduoduo is a highly criticised online shopping platform that you must never ever speak of on social media, because people will slam you for promoting sweat shops, etc.

Temu has a reputation for undelivered packages, mysterious charges, incorrect orders, and unresponsive customer service. It's been subject to over 4,000 complaints to the U.S. Better Business Bureau and has a BBB customer rating of less than 1.5 stars.[68]

But I don't care, do I, because I want socks with hearts on them for seventy cents. Who cares if they skim your credit card and send the details and your home address to some offshore killers! Who cares if the packages don't arrive – they cost a sprinkle of crumbs! Who cares if you live or die!

But it's not just socks. What else does Temu sell, you ask? The better question, my friend, is what does Temu not sell?

Over the past few months I have bought twenty-cent razor holders for the shower, a kitchen spray bottle identical to one you could buy at Father Rabbit (for about a hundred times the price), Vivie's chicken Halloween costume, fridge organisers, Xbox controller neon signs for the boys' playroom, a rug, a little tray table that clips onto the couch arm, a marble tray for my jewellery, a rubbish bin for my car and about a trillion other things. I've spent hundreds and hundreds of dollars yes, but all on bargains. Thousands of dollars' worth of absolute tat.

Temu also offers scammer opportunities to earn credits through spin-the-wheel games or referrals, but you must always spend a hundred dollars to earn these credits, and you will also lose friends who look at your invitations to sign up and think – rightly so – that you are tragic. A petrol station worker recently pleaded with a friend of mine to use his referral code to sign up so he could get a discount. This is the grip Temu has on the nation.

Earlier this year, *Saturday Night Live* dropped a video parodying the e-commerce platform with a bogus ad for 'Xiemu'. In the since-gone-viral clip, models prance across the screen in ten-dollar dresses and five-dollar shoes as a voice-over proclaims, 'How so cheap? Don't worry about it! No prisoners involved! Normal number of working hours each week!' And after Jake Gyllenhaal incurs a nosebleed after sniffing his supposedly lead-free button-down, the voice-over insists, 'No lead!'

But I don't care about lead, do I? Because the easiest and most addictive way to get a powerful and fast serotonin hit is adding twenty-seven twenty-seven-cent things to my cart at 2 a.m. and clicking Submit Order.

Temu packages arrive at my house literally every second or third day. Stu is irate at my compulsive Temu-ing, but I try to assuage his concerns, shrieking, 'It's fine!! Everything is so cheap!!' He explains that everything is not so cheap because when I am buying one trillion things for twenty-seven cents it actually adds up to twenty-seven trillion dollars.

I ignore him though, don't I? Because packages.

Packages arriving at my door, addressed to 'Sinead Corcoran Dye, and no husband or children,' bring me both a joy and serenity that no exercise class (if I was ever able to take one) or meditation ever could.

Don't know what to buy? You do not need to. Temu will tell you what you need. Temu will light the way.

Putting things in my calendar

Anything, doesn't matter. Book a manicure for next week and put that in. Put in 'might take laxatives on Tuesday 'cause have that work lunch and will likely be bloated and thoroughly relish having diarrhoea for the after-effect of feeling reborn.' Honestly put anything in – it's not the thing you put in that helps, it's the putting in of it. I think because it must tell your brain 'See, you will get through this, look – you have many things pencilled in for next week when you will definitely be alive, not dead, and things will be much better by then, you'll see.'

Clean pajamas

Even if it's 6 p.m. and you're still in the same pajamas from the night before, just shower and put on freshies. If you're sleeping in your Junkie Bed™, don't worry about finally doing the sheets tonight, just do pajamas – much less effort required. There's always tomorrow for sheets. A new dawn, a new day.

Getting low on the ground

Honestly fuck the rest of yoga, like no thank you, but truly that child pose thing does work. I do it about five times a day – make my potato-shaped body as compact as possible and smoosh my forehead into the ground. I'm no medical expert, obviously, but I've decided it works because the smaller you are (and closer to hell where you belong, maybe?) the safer you feel.

As many duvets as you own, all piled on top of you
So you are on the brink of suffocation but still A-OK.

Swinging
Not the sexual kind – as my thinking is what would be more anxiety-inducing than an orgy (in case you are left out and no one wants you and you end up just in a corner alone giving the other guests encouraging 'doing great!' nods and smiles? And when I say 'my thinking,' I mean I literally fret over this scenario daily and wonder how I would ever emotionally recover from it).

Anyway, I mean the swinging on the swings at the playground type of swinging.

I discovered this one day in lockdown during one of my furious lockdown walks. I sat briefly on a local swing set to doomscroll Instagram and absent-mindedly found myself swing-swing-swaroo. And it was absolutely divine?

I swing-swing-swarooed back and forth in utter rapture, as a rush of calmness washed over me and my heart filled with joy – pausing only briefly to put my EarPods in and turn my head away when a mum asked me if her toddler could have a turn – and I swing-swing-swarooed some more.

I later learned that studies show the gentle back-and-forth motion of swinging activates the parasympathetic nervous system, which basically tells your body to chill out and stop being a hysterical banshee.[69] This movement also stimulates brain areas that release serotonin, a neurotransmitter that smashes anxiety to death!! The rhythm of swinging also helps distract the mind, offering some much-needed respite from stress/the banshee wails.

Not just for hoots, swings have been shown to improve emotional regulation in children, particularly those with autism or sensory sensitivities – which is why therapy swings are now a thing you can buy, and I want one so bad.

Also, studies have shown that vestibular stimulation, such as rocking or swinging, can promote deeper and more restful sleep in both children and adults because the gentle rocking motion activates the raphe system of the brain which relaxes the body and gets it nice and snoozy.[70] This is why babies who are gently rocked fall asleep more rapidly than ones who are (gently) flung in their cots while the flinger says, 'See ya, friend, na-night'.

Depending on how the day has gone, I am either a rocker or a flinger. We strive to be rockers every day obviously but some days we do not have the rocks within us. But that's okay, there's always tomorrow, Mum.

Watching blackhead videos

Need I say more? Okay I will but surely this is not even necessary because it's not like I'm some outlier freak. Because right now as you read this, in trillions of other bedrooms around the globe, a trillion members of the cult-like following who have pledged their lives to Dr Pimple Popper (AKA Sandra Lee) are currently balls-deep in watching someone's pumpkin-sized shoulder cyst be exploded by black-gloved hands – and these devout cult members are having to muffle their hisses of delight while their mentally sound partner sleeps next to them.

According to scientists, popping your own pimples releases the happy-go-lucky chemical, dopamine, in your brain, and that combined with the cathartic rollercoaster of something disgusting or 'dangerous' building up and then subsiding – there is nothing more mwah. It is like edging, but for the brain.

I absolutely insist you watch the clips with the sound off, so you can properly be aroused by the build-up and experience the final detonation without any spoilers that the climax is near – while you're nothing short of delirious by constantly somersaulting between overwhelming nausea and pure glee.

But don't limit yourself to being just a mere content consumer! I urge you to empower yourself to be your own Dr Pimple Popper, like I have. Each and every night after we've put the children to bed, I fetch my (definitely not) hermetically sealed instrument tray of 'tools'. This includes stock-standard nail files, clippers, cuticle scissors and tweezers and also my never-sterilised-between-uses metal hooks, comedone extractors, needles, blackhead remover stabbing prongs and literal scalpels (only stopping short of an authentic dentist drill) – all of which, surely, should not be available for public purchase.

I then gently announce to my patient (Stu) that 'we're ready for him now,' and lie him down on the couch while he whimpers.

'It's time for your surgery! Don't be afraid, you're in safe hands,' I smile.

As I don't currently have access to any proper sedation – beyond clonazepam, and I am not sharing those – the patient is awake for the procedures which often makes things difficult as he thrashes around. But I'm an old hand at this point, so I know to just pin him down with my knees while we continue with the extraction procedures.

What are we extracting you ask? Just anything really, literally anything goes! Ingrown hairs, regular outgrown hairs that are just going about being hairs and minding their own business, earwax, stuff under toenails, stuff deep inside the bellybutton recesses, blackheads, whiteheads, anyheads – we don't see colour, we are all one.

And once annually, under the guise of 'if you actually loved me, you would let me, I only ask for this one thing,' I manage to convince Stu to do BabyFoot.

If you have not heard of BabyFoot, prepare to finally start living your life the way God intended you to. It's a Japanese foot-peel product which consists of two plastic foot-shaped bags filled with freezing cold liquid that resembles spit but is actually glycolic and lactic acids that eat away at your calluses.

Directions instruct you to simply dip your feet into these arctic spit bags and schlep around the house in them for approximately one hour before removing and rinsing.

Then: absolutely nothing happens. This is the (only) worst part about BabyFoot – the immediate aftermath is very anticlimactic.

But then around nine to eleven days later – when you've long forgotten all about those spit bags – you'll be out a bar, feel an odd sensation in your heel, subtly slip your shoe off and scream. Your foot will resemble a colony of snakes that have shed themselves five hundred times over and then withered and died.

If you're normal, you will cancel all social plans that require open-toed shoes and wait for the skin to naturally detach. If you're like me, you will cancel all social plans so you can stay home and feverishly peel the layers off with tweezers while sending photos of the skin piles to your long-suffering loved ones.

You will again pin your partner down with force so you can rip his layers off too, while he begs for mercy, pleading for you to 'just not tear against the grain.' But tearing against the grain is the only path to the holy place of true rapture.

You will then be hurt, confused and angry as to why your partner is insisting you throw the piles of dead skin away instead of 'saving them.' Like they, as they always do, saved you.

Design stuff on Canva with no rhyme and for no reason

If you have not heard of Canva, it's a graphic design software platform where, with the help of fancy templates, in just three clicks non-artsy plebs can razzle up a quite-impressive brochure or birthday card and pretend they are a qualified and experienced graphic designer.

You can create literally anything and everything and it does not matter if you'll never use it. During my most recent mental breakdown I fashioned some paintball invites for my stepson's birthday party, which did not exist, and next breakdown I'm thinking I might dive into colour swatch and font pairings for my own funeral programme.

Laughing At Your Enemies

This is me and Stu's favourite pastime of all. And we don't just do it when I'm unwell – we do it when I'm weller than well and it makes me the wellest!

Laughing At Your Enemies consists of looking people up on Instagram who used to be in your life but no longer are – think ex-boyfriends, ex-friends, high-school bullies – and inspecting their photos for physical flaws, such as a hair out of place or a minor gap between their front teeth, and cackling cruelly. That's it. That's the entire activity.

Talking to yourself like you're five

I always try to do this as much as possible in the kind, gentle, validating, empathetic and compassionate way we reserve for children while we constantly berate ourselves, but I also mean re-parenting yourself the next time you're spiralling, too.

Just like the Genie popping out of the lamp in Aladdin, Mum (you) is going to pop out at the next scheduled spiral, yoohoo! And the Genie Mum's going to say, 'Hmm, poor wee saus, what do we need here?' She (you) will probably say responsible and wise things like, 'You're allowed four TikTok videos before bed, then no more screen time,' or, 'You can't just have a box of Shapes for dinner, you need to eat at least one green thing,' or, 'Okay, you can have ONE glass of wine, but no more than that because you need a decent sleep tonight,' and you'll probably be like, 'Wait, aren't I five?' And Mum will say, 'Oh yeah. Well maybe we are French parents and one with dinner is okay.' You'll nod your head and say, 'Yes Mum,' and follow the rules then brush your teeth, read a quick story before bed and lights off. You might even say, as my mum used to say to me, 'Everything will be brighter in the morning.'

Because even mums need to be mummed sometimes, especially

when their own mum isn't around – and especially when they're sick.

Sometimes, even my special personalised list of Tool Things only helps alleviate an episode a little bit if it's really bad, so I have to just try to stay calm and wait it out. A 'good' episode typically lasts a few hours, an average one a couple of days and a really bad one can last two weeks. Then eventually I'll start to sober up, until the next one.

But I now try with all my might to think of my illness like another physical one that has flare-ups, like hay fever or migraines. I try to think, *I wouldn't be frightened if it was hay fever or migraines*, not, *Maybe it's never going to stop, maybe I'm stuck like this forever*. I try to remember the only thing that is forever is nothing.

When it's bad, though, it's still bad. Even though it's better now, and I'm so much better than I was at managing it, I will have to manage it for the rest of my life. And when it is bad, while not terrifying, it still impacts my day-to-day, like having to make an excuse to a new mum friend as to why I can't drive over the Harbour Bridge for coffee. Or having to get Stu to carry the baby up the stairs because I'm scared I'll drop her, because I can't feel her in my hands.

I try not to think about whether a cure is coming, or if I'll somehow cure myself. I try not to think about it all as much as I can, because when I don't think about it, DPDR rarely visits me. I think maybe that's because the monster thinks, *Oh well I won't bother with her if she's just going to fucking ignore me*. In the meantime, I'm eternally grateful to Stu, who looks after me when I'm sick (and even when I'm not sick – just all the time), my friends who check in on me and the public mental-health system. It is an underfunded system that cops a lot of criticism, but I genuinely believe I wouldn't be here today if it weren't for the staff at the Taylor Centre who stayed with me on the phone that night on my balcony. The frontline staff do so much with so little, and with one in five adults being diagnosed with a mood and/or anxiety disorder, we need it now more than ever.

As a former dating columnist, I've been writing about my personal life for the better part of a decade, but when I decided to go public with this illness a few years ago – in the hopes it might raise awareness for a very rare condition – I was really apprehensive about sharing my story. While society is now much more accepting of mental illness, it still felt terrifying – and career-limiting – to write about it for public consumption. But at the time I decided that if it shed some light on a frightening illness that's relatively unknown, or it made one person with DPDR feel less alone, then I was doing something good.

14 FEBRUARY 2013, 10:47 A.M.

Sinead Corcoran has posted to Facebook

'Hey everyone! It's not too late to join our glam Fun Run team this weekend and raise money for the NZ Breast Cancer Foundation <3 <3 <3'

5 likes, 3 comments.

Michele: How does one join the team?

Sinead: You are already on the team.

Michele: Yes, but what about the hordes of others who would just love to join us??

I don't want to rule the world

Dear Vivie,

Last weekend I went into the city to meet up with friends for drinks, because your Aunty George was over from Sydney for the weekend. But after two wines I made my apologies, kissed Aunty G and fled. She understood, because I was a week away from this book deadline so I could not afford to have a big Saturday night and be written-off the next day. Also, I don't really go out on the weekend anymore.

G came over from Sydney the summer right after you were born, too. And while your dad looked after you, I partied every night right through Christmas and New Years. This is unfathomable to me now; I don't know how I did this – or why I wanted to.

But I think it's probably because I had suffered so much for nine months and had been clawing at the walls for any semblance of fun – so when I wasn't pregnant anymore, maybe I was trying to make up for lost time and gorge myself at the buffet because I'd starved myself for so long.

I never knew why people said going out partying on the weekend just isn't worth it anymore when you've got to look after kids the next day. Like, yeah, it's shit having to wrangle a baby when you're hungover, but it's definitely doable – just put them in front of Ms. Rachel?

But then I think maybe I grew up a bit, or a lot, and realised that when I already miss out on so much time with you because I'm working – and now more than ever with this book – my weekends with you are most precious.

There's just no night out that would ever be worth not being one hundred per cent for you the next day, or too tired to enjoy you. I've had nearly twenty years of nights out, and I don't think there's anything out there I haven't seen or done already a million times.

So, most Friday and Saturday nights, I'll stay in with you so that in the morning I can see everything you see, and see everything you do and do it all with you. And I want to do that almost every weekend for as long as you want to hang out with me. (I only say almost 'cause occasionally me and Dad really should have a night away so we have a shot at not getting divorced. Which is in your best interests.)

I will not lie to you though; I do drink during the week. Most nights I drink exactly one point five glasses of wine at approximately 5:15 p.m. This is also entirely in your best interests because if I didn't, I fear one of those nights I really might just pack up the car and drive off into the sunset and leave the lot of you behind. Because every night in this house is the first *Saw*.

You will not be familiar with the *Saw* movie franchise (because both your father and I hate horror movies – just as I feel about rollercoasters or Spookers theme park, why would you pay money to be traumatised when life is traumatising enough for free?) unless you're eleven as you read this, which would mean Poppa has already made you watch all ten of the *Saw* movies with him, like he did with me, and Poppa will now be paying for your therapy.

But if you happen to have avoided this mentally maiming binge fest, *Saw* goes like this: the main character, Jigsaw, has clearly Been Through Some Stuff and is now absolutely cooked in the head, and dresses as a puppet and rides a tricycle. Jigsaw is very passionate about cycling and also putting the world to rights – and making sure people learn their lessons when they've done some bad bits and bobs. But instead of sending them to some sort of wellness retreat or rehab, he puts them in intricate traps and lets them decide how far they're willing to go to save their own lives – with the hope this experience will teach them the value of life.

As your mother, I will not elaborate on what these traps entail. I will simply say this: remember how anxiety-inducing that board game Mouse Trap is as you wait for the little plastic hatch to slide down the stick and catch the mouse? Well, *Saw* is a bit worse than that.

Anyway, every night at approximately 5:45 p.m., I hear a faint clickety clack sound approaching. Is it the reaper, finally here to take me away? No. It's much worse. It's the clickety clack of three wheels. And my blood runs cold. Because I know what that sound means.

Clickety clack. Clickety clack. Clickety clack.

And into the lounge wheels your oldest brother, Jigsaw, pedalling on his trike. And he's smiling. But it's the smile of a sadist.

'Would you guys like to play a game?'

The Sausage Game was invented by your brothers. The rules are simple: you just ask each other inane questions and answer only by saying the word 'sausage', but here's the kicker – you must do it without smiling or laughing. Which seems to be near-impossible if you are a child or a person not utterly devoid of energy and joy. As an exhausted mother, this is the easiest game in the world for me. This is one singular piece of piss.

The game usually looks something like this:

'What was in Vivie's nappy when you changed her earlier?' Jigsaw will ask me through sniggers.

'Sausage,' I'll respond with dead eyes and gritted teeth.

'What do your farts smell like?'

'Sausage,' I choke out.

'Ugh, Sinead won again.'

Because unless I've had one point five wines, I have never lost The Sausage Game. And I never will. Because I hate it here. And as it's transpired, this game does not work on me because instead of teaching me the value of life, I crave the sweet release of death.

But after one point five red wines, I love The Sausage Game. I shriek with cackles; I lose every time. So thank you Jigsaw, you have shown me how far I'm willing to go to save my own life, and the lives of my children. And that is fifteen centimetres down a bottle of wine.

When I was leaving the bar last weekend to come home to write this book, I felt so bad, because G was only over for that one weekend and I barely got a chance to talk to her. I shouted, 'Keep me posted on where you guys end up! I'll try to come back after I get Vivie to bed!' My friend Chloe, who is also a mum, said, 'No you will not!' and I said, 'I will, I will definitely try to come back!' but I did not try one iota, because I had to write this book and I wanted to be fresh for you in the morning and, also, I simply could not be fucked going back out.

I think people use 'try to' all the time when they really cannot be fucked going to something and ninety-nine per cent of the time this phrase is used is when it is a friend's BYO birthday dinner. Because, yes, on paper, how wonderful to have all your friends from all walks of life and all corners of the Earth come together as one to celebrate the shining star that you are who lights up every room, and break bread at a Thai restaurant with four-dollar corkage? Absolutely divine.

If you have never heard of such an event, thank fuck for you, because that means someone somewhere outlawed them and not a moment too soon, in fact many moments too late.

What actually transpires? This gaggle of complete strangers

who they've collected in their travels through life are all shoved around a table, and the one person you know has somehow ended up down the other end. So, you get stuck sitting next to the birthday girl's former colleague, which you established within the first seven seconds of sitting down when you asked, 'So how do you know the birthday girl?' and they said, 'Oh we used to work together!' and you said, 'nice!' and then there was simply nothing else to be said.

The truth of the matter is that it doesn't matter how beloved you are by your gaggle, no one can be fucked making small talk with a stranger at the end of a long week. But all of these birthday girls still insist on these BYO dinners and I can't understand it 'cause, Hey birthday girl, remember two weeks ago when it was our other friend's birthday and she made us go to a BYO dinner, and you were texting me under the table saying, 'This is so fucking shit, why do people do these'?

Maybe this is part of the reason I don't really drink much anymore. Because at least four times a year for the past fourteen years, I have been forced to endure these birthday dinners. And the only way that is humanly possible is by drinking a minimum of one point five bottles of sour Woolworths Chardonnay (which you will later vomit up in the restaurant bathroom that has a floral curtain instead of a door, along with the bland Pad Thai you consumed that tastes like that Maggi pouch pasta everyone's mum cooked in the 90s.)

But at every one of these dinners, there will be a minimum of four empty chairs. And this is because these four people, they are not just pretty faces – oh no, no. They are sharp as a tack. They are the wiliest of foxes. They are always one step ahead. These four people, they messaged the birthday girl earlier in the week, saying that they are so snowed under at work and their grandma just died and also their dog and their dog's grandma too – but that they will 'definitely, definitely try to make it!'

So I'm not going to tell you all the things I will try to get right as your mum, Vivie. Because this BYO dinner thing has ruined the word 'try' for me. It's become this Get Out of Jail Free card for if you can't be bothered.

Instead of saying what I'll try to do, I'm going to say what I really *want* to do. So that you know if sometimes I don't get all of these things right all of the time, and if sometimes I can't get to you because I'm tied up writing, it's not because I didn't want to. Believe me, every time I wanted to – more than everything else.

And I know this is insane, but right now I want to be back in the clinky linky with you, because it was small and it was quiet and life was so simple. In the clink I just slept. Then you woke up, so I woke up. I changed you and fed you a bottle. You went back to sleep. I made a new bottle. I thought of your dad. I went back to sleep. There was nothing else to do, so I had nothing to do, so I did nothing. And because the only things inside that room beside a bed and your cot were you and me.

Life is not so simple right now.

This morning you were still asleep when I had to leave to go to work. And then when I came home I had about ten minutes of Quality Time with you before I had to go and finish this book. Except you didn't know that was our allocated Quality Time window, because you're just a baby, so when I tried to pull you into my lap for a cuddle you squirmed away to have Quality Time with the cat – which involves you stabbing him with felt-tip pens.

Then I missed out on giving you dinner and a bath and putting you to bed because I was writing. I knew you were fine with your dad, but I don't feel fine not being with you. And every day right now is the same as today, until I finish the book. And I know this is all temporary, but I'm just so tired. And today your brother told me that this morning when I'd left for work you stood up by yourself for the first time and I didn't see it. I saw you do everything when it was just me and you in the clink.

But I promise I'm nearly finished the book, and I don't want to have a night out to celebrate. All I want is to give you dinner and a bath and put you to bed, and to not have to have an allocated

Quality Time window – just have Any Time, All The Time.

So, if you don't feel like hanging right now and, instead, you're in the mood for violating the cat, you go for it! Catch ya on the flip, see ya round the traps – I'm actually thinking of swinging by the kitchen in an hour or so if you're 'round, but if I see ya I see ya, no sweat.

There are other things I want.

I want to keep writing to you. Right now, I'm going to say for the next wee while this writing will be of the simple but effective 'luv ya 😊' on a Post-it note variety – because, not sure if you're aware, I just wrote an entire book for you and I'm really running out of both steam and content here. But I promise when I've got fresh juice in the tank and my hands have recovered from being RSI-riddled, withered chicken claws from typing 85,000 words, I will write you proper letters.

I wish my mum had written me letters.

About her, and about me, and about everything she wished she'd told me – and everything she wished she'd be around to tell.

Stories about me growing up, stories about how I was going to grow up.

The life she imagined I'd have, who I'd grow up to be and that she knew, whoever that was, I would be just right.

Everything she loved most about me, all the special things that make me me.

And how much I meant to her. How I was her whole world, and how she wished she could stay.

I asked her to, and I know she tried because she told me she was trying. And maybe that's another reason I hate the word. Because she might have tried, but I didn't get a letter.

She was so sick and tired by then – and how was she meant to wrap up all of those things into a letter and say it all right? Especially when something I was going to read at twenty-two wouldn't read the same when I was thirty-two, and it wouldn't answer all the different questions I have now. Especially now I'm a mum.

It makes me so, so sad that I don't have a letter – but I'm not mad, because I know she wanted to write me one.

I bet she *wanted* to be able to think about and write about everything she wished she'd told me and everything she wished she'd be around to tell me. And I bet she *wanted* to say she wished she could stay. But I bet she couldn't even let herself think of me, and everything she loved most about me, and all the special things that make me *me*. Because it would hurt so much and make her feel so sick. And she was already so sick, Viv.

On top of all of that, she wasn't a writer, like I am, so it would have been even harder for her to do it.

I'm currently writing this while I lie horizontally across the bed with my laptop on its side so I can try to read whatever garbage I'm typing. I'm drenched in sweat with my head hanging over the edge because we've all got gastro the week my book is due – of course. And every time I finish a paragraph, I lean over and vomit into a bucket then write some more.

While I was too sick to work my whole pregnancy, what I could manage was a tiny monthly column about you. Most of those columns were written in hospital, on a laptop on its side, tangled up with IV wires. I couldn't rest it on my belly because there were machines hooked up to it, monitoring you because your heart would go too fast sometimes when we were both dehydrated. And I'd hang over the edge of the bed every time I finished a paragraph to vomit into a bucket then write some more.

If my mum was reading this right now, she'd say, 'Oh colour me surprised – here Sinead goes again, comparing her gastro and hyperemesis to my terminal cancer, yes we are indeedy fighting the same battle!' But what I'm trying to say is that I'm a writer, and even when it's hard it's still easy for me because this is what I'm meant to do. And it's even easier when I'm writing for you.

I bet what I write for you is probably pretty similar to what my mum would have written for me if she could. So, I can write for her and write for me and write for you, easy peasy.

I want to write you letters throughout your whole life that you can keep forever and read whenever you want. I want to write so many that you'll always have something to look forward to. Like an advent calendar that isn't just twenty-five days long, but goes for the rest of your life and you can open a new window anytime.

I want to be there for everything – big or tiny – that ever happens in your life, and be able to get to wherever you are so I don't miss a single thing. If I'm not there, you don't have to pretend like I'm there when I'm not – it's not the same and it hurts. You can be mad, and you can be sad, and I'll get it.

I never want you to be the last one left when I come to pick you up from daycare, school or anywhere else. I want to get you home as soon as possible so we don't have to have a Quality Time window, we can just have Any Time, All The Time.

But most of all I want you to know how very wanted you were. Even every day of those nine months. And even when we had to go to the clinky linky – you were the Most Wanted criminal.

My mum couldn't write, but she could run. And just like how I don't just write, I'm a writer – she didn't just run, she was a runner. Every morning of my entire life I would wake up and she would be in the kitchen, panting and sweating and freezing. She would be freezing because she'd go running in the middle of the night, in the dark, so that she'd be home in time for when I woke up. Even after she got cancer and became really sick, she still ran through the nights.

Not only am I not a runner, I cannot run, but more crucially – I do not want to run.

If you ever happen to see me running somewhere, run for your fucking life because it means I'm being chased by someone with a knife and I am running for my life. And I'd honestly run about twenty metres and then just say, 'ahh nah can't be bothered, just get it over with' and let myself be killed.

I did run once though. A few months before my mum died, me, Annabel and Em signed up to take part in some Breast Cancer fun run thing – obviously in part 'for my mum' but mostly so we could Instagram it so everyone knew we were really good people, you know?

My mum announced she was going to run too. And we were like 'Michele, you cannot do a fun run. You are literally a dead woman walking. You cannot be a dead woman running because you'll collapse and all these kids will trip over this dead body and suddenly the run will probably not be the most fun these kids have ever had.'

But she would not be dissuaded so we were like, 'Fuck's sake, this is going to be like a Round The Bays *Weekend At Bernie's*,' dragging this bitch along Tamaki Drive.

When we got to the starting line, we said to her sternly, 'You take it easy, do you hear us!? Under no circumstance are you to run! Ambling only!'

And she saluted and said, 'Yup, understood!'

Then the whistle blew and she blasted off like the old bat out of hell that she was. And we spent the entire fun run having not so much fun because we were trying to run while also trying to locate a corpse on the ground. But we didn't find a corpse, and we didn't catch her until hours later when we found her standing by a hedge eating a Bunnings sausage, with a medal around her neck because Bernie The Bat had come first in the entire race. FIRST. Because she was a runner. So even when it was hard, it was still easy for her, because that was what she was meant to do.

I can't remember exactly when she went for her very last run – but I know it was unfathomably close to the end. Even for the best runner, that one would not have been easy. But I know with absolute certainty, that she ran as hard as she could, for as long as she could.

Your dad was watching some Man Alone Seeking Vengeance in Space shit last night before we went to bed, and I wasn't really watching but I made the colossal mistake of asking him what it was about, and also how does space actually work you know?

And he tried to explain it all to me, but eventually I had to put my head between my knees and make him stop because actually I've realised I can't talk about this universe stuff 'cause it's too big for my brain to comprehend and makes me want to throw up. But what I got from Dad before I nearly passed out was this:

Heat from the sun makes Earth warm enough to live on, and without light from the sun there would be no plants or animals and, therefore, no food – and the Earth would freeze and die.

We orbit the sun because it's so big it has a strong gravitational pull. And now I'm lying here with my head over this sicko bucket and I'm thinking of my mum and I miss her, and I'm thinking how she was my sun and I was the Earth.

And now I'm thinking that I want it to be different for you. That I'm going to make it different for you.

I am still your sun, but you are not the Earth.

I am your sun because I will keep you tethered to the ground so you don't ever spin out into the abyss. And the tether will be so strong that it will always keep you safe and keep you tethered to yourself and your body. You won't float far away from yourself like I sometimes do.

I am your sun because my whole job is to keep you warm. But, Vivie, you are not my sun.

I am yours, but I think I also used to be something else I read about.

That eighty light years from Earth, there have been sightings of rogue planets, floating all alone. They are not gravitationally bound to any star. So, they wander the Milky Way alone without a parent star.

And it's not clear whether these are orphaned planets or failed stars.[71]

I know it's very depressing, sorry, but stay with me.

Instead of relying on one source – the sun – these rogue planets survive from the light of lots of little stars instead.

That's how I've survived, Viv.

I think my mum just wanted us to be our own little solar system.

Just the sun and the Earth following her around and around. So, when my sun died and the only thing keeping me warm was gone and the only thing keeping me tethered had broken off, I wandered alone in the dark for a long time.

I don't anymore.

It's been warm and it's been light again for a long time now because of your dad and your brothers and all the people in the back of this book who keep me tethered so strong and so tight.

I am your sun, and I will keep you warm and that is one of my jobs. But my other job is collecting all those other little stars for you, your backup generators. I am collecting them because I will not let you be the Earth who needs the sun to survive.

My friend Lia says that when you don't feel like climbing into my lap for a cuddle and instead you push me away, it's a good thing. I do such a good job of showing you that when you need me, I am always, *always* here, so most of the time you don't need me. She says a kid who doubted a mother's love would never squirm off their mum to stab the cat with pens, because they would be scared that their mum wouldn't be there when they turned around.

You're only a year old and I have already collected you so many stars.

I will never be the sole thing that keeps you warm and keeps you tethered. You will have so many stars to lean on. I will make sure your entire universe is not just me.

I will make it so big that you can't even comprehend it.

Love,
Mum x

23 AUGUST 2014, 2:36 P.M.

Michele: A youngish nurse man just came in

Sinead: Is he good looking y/n

Michele: I will find my glasses so I am prepared next time he comes in so that I can confirm

Sinead: OK let me know urgently before I come in looking like a rodent

Michele: Speaking of, you know who has improved with age? Justin Timberlake. He is starting to look less weaselly

Sinead: It's so unfortunate you will not be given the same chance at redemption

Michele: I know. Also, I got Chris to shave the back of my neck before we came here and the haircut produced a segment of fluff the size of a ten-cent piece. It would have had to have been the world's smallest haircut

Sinead: LMAO

Michele: (^^^)

Michele: 🐧

Michele: Just trying some things out

Michele: You see my penguin?

Sinead: Yes, busy day for you then

Michele: What time do you finish nannying?

Sinead: 12 and it's so fucking cold

Michele: Set fire to the children

Sinead: HAHAHHA

Sinead: When I finish should I come get you and we go to the movies?

Michele: I can't now honey. It's too much effort.

Sinead: That's OK.

Sinead: I'm just a bit sad today. Annabel's gone out for lunch with her mum and I just feel sad because we can't anymore.

Michele: I know. I'm so sorry to make you sad. But hey at least we've had lots of lunches.

Sinead: Yeah

Michele: Lots and lots.

Sinead: I know. Hundreds.

Michele: What time are you coming in?

Sinead: I'll come as soon as I finish

Michele: Okay just wanted to make sure I'd be here haha

Sinead: What do you mean, where would you go???

Michele: Yah that's why it's funny

Sinead: AHAHHAHA

Dear Sinead, I'm back baybay!

HEY, IT'S ME! ME AS IN YOU! I'M BACK BABY!

So, I finished writing this book months ago and it's Vivie's eighteen-month birthday right now. And all of a sudden out of nowhere my baby went somewhere and now there's a whole big girl toddler here instead.

(Also, before I had her, I never got why mums would be like 🥰'sHe's 158 wEeks oLd'🥰 like, just say your kid is three, you loser? But now I get it. It's because one week your baby is just a boring blob sucking their own feet, and then a week later they're playing scrabble and baking profiteroles. It makes more sense to go by weeks – a week is a lot in baby blob time.)

Anyway, so it's me from the future I guess; I have returned to you in the DeLorean, and I have a message for you, for reals. And you know this message has got to be good, right? Because if it wasn't, there wouldn't be a shot in hell I would return to the constant power-chuck-inducing stress of writing a book as long as I live (but

Kate, my publisher, if you're reading this, yes I'll do another for many money).

Anyway. The message to past me. Here we go.

So right now, Vivie has just turned one, right? Well, brace yourself cause something even more huge is about to happen for you. Something you never would have believed would happen to you ever again.

Four years ago, two weeks into starting a brand-new job in an attempt to find something that wouldn't make you sick, you were so sick that you crashed your car. And that's when you knew this would be your last brand-new job. As you walked out of your brand-new job's office door for the last time, you knew there and then that the door had well and truly slammed closed on your big sparkly career too. The last sequin left, of all the sequins that had peeled off over the last four years, that last one dropped off onto the ground when that office door swung shut. And the name I'd spent a decade building for myself, that name in shining lights – well the lights were off now. And I was just a nobody in a dark room with dirty stepped-on sequins all over the floor.

But guess what. I know you've been in that dark room for a few years now – and you've even gotten used to it. Actually, you love it in there. Because it's small and it's quiet, kinda like the clink. And it's just you in there so no one knows if you make a mistake, so you can't ever get in trouble, so you're never afraid, so you're never sick, so you're always safe. But very soon there's going to be a knock on your little dark door. And someone's going to ask you to come outside again where it's big and it's light and it's loud, and they're going to offer you your first new job since your last new job.

And you'll be so fucking scared.

But then you'll decide you're going to be so fucking brave. Because you don't want Vivie to have a scared mum who's too scared to do scary things. You want Vivie to have a scared mum who's so scared to do scary things but then says. 'Okay, I'll try. I'll try for Vivie.'

And guess what. This first new job since your last new job won't make you sick. Maybe because it's a better job, or maybe because you're better now – because you got yourself better. Or maybe it's both. Whatever it is, this new job won't make you sick and you won't crash your car and you won't have to leave after only two weeks. And I know that because as I write this to you now, I've just gotten home from work – from that first new job since your last new job. Except it isn't new anymore – it's just my job.

But hey, you know how I just said maybe you're better now? You are, I promise. You're much better now, nearly all of the time. Sometimes you still have little wobbles, like everyone does. But unfortunately, as we know, you're different to everyone, so these little wobbles make you get a little bit sick again – sometimes a lot sick. And I'm so sorry to have to tell you this, but very soon the ground's going to start shaking beneath your feet.

Why, though? Why now? You're doing good! You're actually doing fucking great thank you! And you'll love your new job and love being a mum and love that you've got a book deal. And yeah, okay, that is a lot to juggle – but you know how to juggle. You learned how to juggle five balls at once when you were six and your mum sent you to a circus holiday programme. You learned to juggle nine balls at once when your mum got sick – your nanny job and uni classes and assignments and exams and looking after a dying mum and trying to be a fun funny clown for her and trying not to cry and trying to stop wishing she'd just die already.

You can definitely juggle it all now, because you have an airtight system. You are a man with a plan. You'll get to spend Quality Time with Vivie in the morning before heading off to work, then leave work early for a whole arvo and even have Quality Time with Vivie again. Then after dinner, bath, bottle and bed-ing her, you'll crack into book writing for an hour before sleepytime – because if you do one chapter a night, you'll easily make your deadline. It's not for ages! See, airtight system. Vacuum packed. Hermetically sealed, baby!

You'll juggle, juggle, juggle and you'll be nailing it and the crowd will cheer. Except then you'll realise – uh oh – a ball is missing.

You're going to drop a ball. A calendar ball.

You're going to forget to keep your eye on that ball. And suddenly, strangely, the calendar ball will say your book deadline isn't ages away, it's a week away.

But that's okay, that's okay! You can do this. You'll just juggle faster, no problem. You'll keep doing that hour of book writing before bed. Except now when you go to bed, you won't take a sleeping pill, take a breather, take it easy. Now you'll take your laptop, take a Red Bull, take a Ritalin. And you'll write all through the night, till it starts to get light. And then you'll get up and go to your work-job and then you'll come home and do your mum-job and then you'll write all through the night again. And you'll do it again the next night and the next night and the next night.

And then – wow, colour you surprised – you'll get fucking sick again.

With migraines. And vomiting. Just like when PND sunk its claws into you all those months ago. And the waves of dissociation that are always looming in the shadows will start to roll in. And some fun new additions to spice it up – all-consuming depression and intrusive suicidal thoughts.

And just like how saying Beetlejuice three times summons that green-haired freak, depression and intrusive suicidal thoughts will also seem to have been conjured to you by a word.

Asha. Asha. Asha.

Remember how Vivie was an early talker – the first baby in our group to say her first word ('hi!') months and months before any of the other kids did?

And you and Stu always assumed Vivie was an early talker and has a big vocab because:

- She has two writers for parents (#nature)
- Who also read nearly her entire bookshelf to her day (Mum) and night (Dad) (#nurture)

You thought it was so cool that she could say cat, ball, car, duck and apple by ten months (even though you have neither taught her this word nor ever given her an apple, so her other mum, Ms. Rachel, must have taught her this one).

And by one year old she could say (a jumbled, basically nonsensical version of) her brothers' names. And Dad, Dadda, Papa and Poppa, her grandad.

But she can't – or won't – say mum, will she? You've spent months and months trying to get her to say it, hours spent pointing at your mouth so she could watch you make the 'muh' sounds. No dice. Can say both her brothers' three-syllable names, and three variations of Dad, is bi-fucking-lingual, but can't say Mum.

And it hurts, I know – and you'll try to push it to the back of your mind and tell yourself it doesn't mean anything. And you'll manage to keep it in the back of your mind most of the time, even when you wobble and you drop the ball and you stop sleeping – right up until one day, out of the blue, Vivie says her daycare teacher's name and not yours.

Asha. Asha. Asha. Asha. Asha. Asha.

Asha, all day – she even picks up your phone and mewls 'Asha!' into it, wanting to hear her talk back.

And then that night when you're getting Vivie ready for bed, the strangest thoughts start seeping into your head, like tendrils of smoke curling up from under a door.

You'll try to brush them off as you brush Vivie's hair, wet from the shower. Because you know brushing her hair always soothes you when you're anxious or out of sorts, which is why you brush her hair about thirty-four times a day. She'll likely be bald by her second birthday.

Stranger still, these thoughts will tell you to try again to get Vivie to say Mum.

So, while you brush her hair, you'll show her how to put her lips together to make the 'mm' noise. And she'll watch you curiously. And then another thought curls up from under the door.

'If she says Mum, that's good – that means she wants you to be her mum, so you're allowed to stay.'

And then more smoke will start to coil around in your head because you've had another thought, that if she doesn't say mum, that means she doesn't want you as her mum. So, you shouldn't be her mum. And you shouldn't actually be here at all.

And then it will get harder to breathe and you'll be trying not to throw up while you show Vivie again how to put her lips together to make the 'mm' noise.

And you'll say 'Vivie, watch Mum. See how she goes "mm"? Mum, Mum, Mum, Mum.

'Say Mum, Vivie. Vivie. Vivie, please say Mum.'

And Vivie will just watch you curiously.

And then Vivie will smile.

And then Vivie will say 'Asha!'

And then it will get so smoky you really won't be able to breathe anymore. And it will be so smoky you won't be able to see her anymore.

I won't lie to you Sin; the next few weeks will be rough. But you will get through, you always do. And you will get better, because remember what I said earlier: I promise you you're so much better now, nearly all of the time.

Yes, from time to time you will have little blips and get sick again, but you will survive them. You always do. Because you've survived much worse.

And you will get the book done – I mean duh, of course you will – you are reading the done book right now.

Oh, and on that Mum thing. Funny story.

One night, not long after that awful night that engulfed you – you'll try to be brave and type 'toddler still won't say mum' into Google's search bar. And you'll brace yourself to be inundated with medical studies and research that says if a toddler Vivie's age still isn't saying Mum it means she's got attachment disorder and has no bond whatsoever with you and never will. And that she doesn't want you (and never will).

And even though you're sure this can't be true, a tiny, paranoid, insecure part of your brain will wonder if maybe you caused it. By being so sick when she was trying to grow inside you, or because when you felt her move in your belly it made you feel nauseous, so you hated her a bit and maybe she knew that – or because sometimes during those nine months you didn't even hate her; it was worse than that. You felt nothing. You didn't feel like her mum, and she didn't feel like your baby and maybe she knew that. Maybe she knew all the times you were so sick that you'd have thoughts that maybe I actually can't do this anymore. Maybe she knew sometimes that you thought about doing the only thing you could have done to end the sickness.

You'll wonder if maybe you caused it when you gave birth, because you were too unwell and too frightened to be awake when they cut her out of you. How could she feel safe with a mum who couldn't even be brave enough to see her be born?

Maybe it's all of that, or maybe it's that you made so many fuck-ups through the first year of her life – too many to count. Or maybe it's because you're a mum who is sick and she can tell, and maybe she wants a mum who is well all the time. Who wouldn't?

Or maybe it's all of the above.

You hit 'enter' on the keyboard.

Google will spit out article after article after article written by medical researchers and paediatricians explaining how newborn infants don't know that their mother is a separate entity to them – instead they believe their mother is a literal extension of themselves, based on Margaret Mahler's theory of separation-individuation.[72] Typically, at around nine months old, babies start to become aware that they are their own person.

The articles will tell you that Dad is usually a baby's first word because 'D' sounds are in a group of consonants that are produced at the front of the mouth, so it's really easy for them to make 'Da' sounds, and that babies often then learn to say their other caregivers' names first because, while they do a lot of the feeding and changing, at some point they leave – so the babies learn how to ask when they're coming back.

While, usually by the time a child is Vivie's age, they are saying mum, occasionally there are exceptions. And, very occasionally, a child even at Vivie's age still doesn't see a distinction between themselves and their mother, because when their mother leaves, if she comes back soon – and her presence is unwavering – the child still subconsciously experiences life through her. And in some cases, if an attachment bond is incredibly strong, the child still thinks their mum is part of them.

A paediatrician friend of mine told me that to an infant a mum is as much a part of them as their feet or hands.

'If they want a drink, they have to say "cup" because their cup tends to disappear, or people put it out of reach. If they want a cookie, they need to say "cookie" because cookies are sometimes available but sometimes not. You're their constant. They know you're always there for them,' she said.

Sometimes they disappear or they're out of reach. Sometimes they're available but sometimes not.

Cat. Ball. Car. Duck. Apple.

Brothers. Dad. Poppa.

Asha.

Things that don't disappear or are never out of reach. Things that are always available.

Feet. Hands.

Mum.

That's why she won't say Mum.

Not because of anything bad you've done or anything you got wrong. It's because of everything good you did and everything you got right.

Vivie still wants to keep Mum.

Acknowledgements

Look I know you are probably thinking ‘omg that book was such a lol’ minus the sad bits obvi that were simply too much, ay!! Like you picked this book up off the shelf being like, ‘Aww, lovely poems on motherhood! Like Jessica Urlichs but a little bit fat!’.

And then you took it home and got a few pages in and you realised you were not in fact reading about little fingers and little toes and you would unequivocally not be able to take a flat lay of one of these gorgeous little sonnets and post it with the TikTok trending sound #IThinkILikeThisLittleLife <3 <3 because you were in fact reading *A Little Life*. <3 <3

But despite the fact that, upon finishing this horrible little tale, Kyle Chandler and his flesh particles all over the walls of Grey Sloan Memorial Hospital (née Seattle Grace) are in better shape than you – I also know you still want to be my friend. Because I am a funny little freak, so everyone thinks I would be such a hoot to have around.

Here is the thing. Do you remember that scene in *Friends* where Ross has just found out about Joey and Rachel and he drinks all the margaritas and he keep telling everyone he's fine and then he squeals EEEEE and does a Mexican jig and then he burns his hands on the fajitas and then through tears says, ‘I'm sorry, it must be the pressure of entertaining.’?

And God how we laff, because it's the second funniest Ross scene of the entire series, second only to PIVOT obviously. But then Joey and Rachel and Charlie leave because he is simply being Too Much and then the episode finishes and God that was a good one. OK, but imagine this is your Real-Life Friend who you made the dire mistake of befriending. And the episode never ends so it's really Too Much now and we're laughing but we are so very very drained.

Which leads me to why I must profusely thank my longest-suffering F.R.I.E.N.D.S who are like, 'Okay you fucking freak, I see you! And we are incredibly exhausted by your company!' And still, all these little plastic ponchos constantly encircle me like a flock of ghostly dementors – knitting together to form one of those huge plastic parachutes, and come rain or shine they shield me from the elements while I dance the Mexican jig.

To my finders, my keepers – Annabelle Borrie, Annabel Herbison, Vanessa Duffy, Clarissa Searle and Meilissa Boderick. For then and for now and for it all from now on.

To Diana Byrne, Chloe Rose, Lia Paddy and in memorium to Georgia Smith, who I asked to read the first draft of this book and she promised she would 'as soon as she got home' and she was so excited. That was nearly eighteen months ago though so I can only assume she never made it home and was sadly slain.

To Shannan Faulker who in 2014 was asked by a friend if they could offload their cat to her because they were moving to London. Except the cat was me and this man was actually not moving anywhere but could Shannan 'please be mates with this girl I'm dating because I need to dump her 'cause she's fucking mental but her mum's about to die and IDK that might be a bad look for me? And you have a dead mum so like, can you take her?'

And she did and I am very grateful because this was pre-Facebook Marketplace so like what was his plan B, would I have been placed into a hessian sack filled with rocks and flung into a river?

To my little mum club. It's still so shit – and it always will be – that they didn't talk about PND in our antenatal class: what not to expect when you're expecting. I still wonder if things might have started out different for me, and for Vivie, if they had. But it wasn't just because of the meds, and because of the mental-health professionals, that it was just a false start, and that's all. They might not have talked, but we did. Big talk, real talk - all through the days and all through those longest nights.

And if ever I went quiet – even just for a day, or did more than one 'sorry I can't make it, so snowed under with the book,' - normal people would say 'no worries, good luck! Xx'. So, I am one of the very, very lucky ones. Because every single time, 'tap tap tap' went the door, and I'd open it to the mums with a snowplough. The guardians of the witching hour, who wouldn't just mark me safe – but make me come out, even just for a minute, to feel the sun and let the warm in.

To Moa Press & Hachette obvi! I am so grateful you gave me this book deal, thank you so much. Like - I was definitely more than content to just leave it at that as I was simply wanting to Instagram the fact that I had been offered a book deal for clout, but okay, wow, you meant actually write it okay cool yay love this!!

My book editor's name is Kate Stephenson, and she's incredible at what she does. But there's also a mum called Kate Stephenson, who happens to be a book editor - and that's the one I really want to thank here. Because at every turn, that mum kept me safe. She never let me wander off, getting so caught up wanting to tell a good story that I forgot after the book ended there would still be a girl, and she wouldn't be able to take the stories back if one day she changed her mind.

Say, a story the girl wrote about how – the truth is - she actually did find a little bit of a start of a letter. And she read it, and it was so, so bad it nearly killed her.

But the girl – me – had an editor that reminded her that the truth is rarely pure and never simple - and that it wouldn't set me free. An editor who never let that truth get in the way of a good story, and who reminded me that the real truth was the girl was so, so sad that she didn't have a letter – but that she knew her mum wanted to write her one.

And when my mum needed to go - another mum always came. Because that's one of the very best things about mums - they can be mums to every little person, even when that little person is all grown up. Especially when they're all grown up – because sometimes, a lot of the time, that's when you need a mum most of all. So, to Caro Meng-Yee, Deborah Pead, Hattie Moleta and Deslie Moffett, who always came.

To Michael Hanly, Emma Clifton, Meisha Kimber and Kirsty Stone, who all played a part – hours and hours of parts - in making this beautiful book cover to hold my whole life, and my mum and Vivie's. Who wanted me to have something so beautiful to look at and to hold because I couldn't hold my mum anymore.

And so, one day I could hold it out and say to my own girl, 'look at what your mum wrote when you were really, really little. And lots of the time even though it was really hard to do, she even wrote it while holding you.'

There were so many days after those longest nights writing when it really did get too hard, though, and I didn't think I could keep going – even when I was unfathomably close to the end. Because even for the best writer – which I am not - a book is not easy.

To Hannah Rorke and Kate Robertson - even though this was really hard to do, I did it because they were always holding me. My two best friends dragged little Bernie junior all the way to the finish line, reminding her the whole way that it was what she was meant to do.

To Ihi Ora (the Taylor Community Mental Health Centre) - in particular Dr Trish van Kralingen in the crisis team, my Key Worker Tom Osborne and Dr Giselle Rausch.

My story of that first dissociative episode which ended on a balcony is eerily similar to the character of Mal's in the film *Inception*, who also lost her grip on reality and became convinced that she was dreaming - teetering on the edge of both sanity and a railing, storeys above concrete. But my story wouldn't end on a balcony, because I had Trish as my totem - tethering me with the firm, unwavering promise that morning would come soon.

In *Inception*, the lookouts watch over the dreamers to ensure they're safe while they sleep – so that even if something goes wrong within the dream or they get trapped in limbo, no harm will come to them in real life. And no harm ever did, because of my lookout Tom – and on the many days after the longest nights I had such a shaky grip on where reality bent and blurred that I couldn't get behind the wheel to get to my appointments, 'tap tap tap' went the door. A watchman of my nightmares, who wouldn't just mark me safe but make me come out, even just for a minute, to feel the sun and let the warm in.

And Giselle who spent the next four years as a dreamcatcher - tirelessly battling the cruel and complex Sandman with a myriad of medications until I woke up – and who wouldn't rest until I could.

To every single person who donates to the Starship Foundation and to all the community groups and organisations like Barfoot & Thompson and Mercury who partner with them to raise much-needed funding to help ensure that children and their families receive the best possible care. One of the life-saving departments that these funds go towards is the MBU.

I wouldn't have this book if I never went to the MBU. And my daughter might not have a mum if it weren't for those donations that went towards paying for enough staff.

But because there were enough that day, one nurse had enough time to see behind one lovely smile and some hollow jokes to what was hiding in plain sight – someone gripping onto a railing as best she could, but she was getting so tired now.

To Vivie's brothers, who are not in this book (much) because I love them too much to tell the truth for a good story.

Say, the one about the 27-year-old who in 2020 seemingly

overnight went from flatting in Ponsonby and Carrie Bradshaw zigging and zagging around town not a care in the world, to blasting down into an apocalyptic pin-sized apartment with two very small war criminals aged six and four.

And despite Jacinda reassuring us that 'if you feel you're in an unsafe environment, you do not need to stay in your home or in your bubble – you can and should leave' and despite the warning from two other now-disgraced world leaders that 'cropped pants make any woman look like a stunted man', that 27-year-old donned her camo trou and helmet and then it was Freak Town population 4! And even now she can still sometimes hear her own screams.

But I didn't mention them (much) because I know everything looks worse written down in black and white – and I can't bear the idea of if one day they read it and read that I found it v difficult at the start, in case that makes them think that they were the absolute pits – when they were just the standard little boy amount of pits.

While I'll always wish my mum hadn't died, there's a quiet comfort in knowing the pain is over now – leaving only rest and peace. I am at last finally free from doing those cursed little Wasgij puzzles she made me do with her, since I could never say 'oh wow, no thank you' because she was about to die, bad look, hadn't met Shannan yet etc. And when they say cancer truly is the cruellest disease, and it impacts the whole family, it's because some lovely nurse told these patients that puzzles are a wonderful and relaxing distraction.

But anyway, these foul little puzzles are beloved for their 'quirky humour and tricky, yet rewarding, challenges' because they come in a box that intentionally has some kind of back-to-front picture on it, so you don't know what the fuck you're doing or where you're going until you get there. And that, my friends, is what we call a metaphor and also an Easter Egg because I did not think who I was meant to be was stepmum, but that bat did! Because Wasgij back-to-front is fucking Jigsaw on his tricycle, isn't it, and I really do love it here, Mum.

My bibliographer's name is Stuart Dye, and he's incredible at what he does. He spent many days and the longest nights re-finding all the links to the proper research in this book, because this is my First Time and I did not know I was meant to keep those for a references section and I couldn't be bothered so I made him do it for zero money.

He also happens to be an editor in real life – and there is simply nothing further to say about that.

Because – to paraphrase another man who looks like a cigarette and is named Hugh Grant – I too consider honesty the most overrated virtue. So, when every time upon finishing one of my chapter drafts Stu posed the question, 'do you mind if I'm honest?' I told him yes, I do.

But my husband is also called Stuart Dye and that's the one I really want to thank here. Because there wouldn't be a book without him. And that's not because there would be no Vivie or because I couldn't write one all by myself. I know I could have, and I would have because I've done lots of things all by myself and this is what I'm meant to do.

It's because this book is so different to everything I've ever written before, and everything I'm known for – which is being funny. And that's because I'm different to who I was before, back when I thought I had to light up every single room so I wouldn't be left alone in the dark again.

I don't need to do that anymore, because he isn't just my home, he's my lighthouse. And on the nights it's still light out, I take our daughter out on the deck in the sun and tilt my cheek up to it. And then tilt it back down, all the way until it rests on her dad's shoulder, and we watch the sun go down.

I've spent so, so many hours this year away from my kids, holed up in my bedroom writing this book. More than I can count. I can't count them because if I do, I'll cry.

I've spent so, so many hours this year not in this room, but with my kids. More than I can count. I can't count them because if I do, I'll cry.

My psychologist's name is Shruti Pathak and she's an incredible psychologist. But there's also a mum called Shruti Pathak who is a psychologist – and that's who I want to thank.

And maybe one day she'll show her kids this part of the book I wrote, and say, 'Hey, I think you'll like this one. It's about your mum – and how lots of the hours she was at work, she was helping another mum, who was really sick, get some rest, and then the other mum got so much better.

'And then that mum went home and went to her room for a little bit to write a book – but very soon she went downstairs to her kids and said HELLO I'M BACK! And the rest of the story is so much better.'

Endnotes

1 Minow, Nell. "Parents' Guide to Bridget Jones's Diary." Common Sense Media, https://www.commonsensemedia.org/movie-reviews/bridget-joness-diary

2 Woodall, Trinny, and Susannah Constantine. 2003. *What Not to Wear*. Riverhead Trade.

3 *Grey's Anatomy*, season 2, episode 16, "It's the End of the World." Directed by Peter Horton. Aired February 5, 2006, on ABC, https://disneyplus.com/; *Grey's Anatomy*, season 2, episode 17, "As We Know It." Directed by Peter Horton. Aired February 12, 2006, on ABC, https://disneyplus.com/.

4 Muru-Lanning, Charlotte. 2023. "The Bitter End of the Grapefruit Fruju." *The Spinoff*, May 3. https://thespinoff.co.nz/kai/03-05-2023/bad-news-for-people- who-love-grapefruit-frujus.

5 Iovine, Vicki. 1999. "Developing a Crush on Your Obstetrician Isn't Unusual." *Los Angeles Times*, May 16. https://latimes.com/archives/la-xpm-1999-may-16-cl-37651-story.html.

6 HER Foundation. n.d. "Postpartum Recovery." https://hyperemesis.org/about-hyperemesis-gravidarum/recovery/.

7 Fenton, Amy, and Ashlie Blakey. 2024. "Mum-to-be, 26, Took Her Own Life After She was Failed in Battle with Debilitating Sickness." *Manchester Evening News*, January 31. https://manchestereveningnews.co.uk/news/uk-news/mum-be-26-took-life-28542160.

8 Jones, Charlie, and Laura Foster. 2023. "Hyperemesis: Scientists Make Pregnancy Sickness Cure Breakthrough." *BBC*, December 14. https://www.bbc. com/news/uk-england-cambridgeshire-67684023..

9 Niven, C. A., & T. Murphy-Black. 2000. "Memory for Labor Pain: A Review of the Literature." *Birth*, 27(4): 244–253. https:// doi. org/10.1046/j.1523-536x.2000.00244.x

10 NZ College of Midwives. n.d. "Birth Trauma." https://midwife.org. nz/women/postnatal/11007-2/

11 Nightingale, Melissa. 2024. "Birth Trauma Affects 50 New Zealand Women Each Day – Mums Share Their Stories." *The New Zealand Herald*, August 10. https://nzherald.co.nz/nz/birth-trauma-affects-50-new-zealand-women-each-day-mums-share-their-stories/SU4PXYIHFBE37F67WMSSR2FYNY/.

12 Ibid.

13 Ibid.

14 Ibid.

15 *Stuff*. 2016. "Adele Lashes Out at Jamie Oliver's New Breastfeeding Campaign." March 28. https://stuff.co.nz/life-style/parenting/baby/breastfeeding/78312986/adele-lashes-out-at-jamie-olivers-new-breastfeeding-campaign

16 Duff, Hilary. 2019. "This One's for the Ladies…" Instagram. May 8. https://instagram.com/p/BxLgOfuAqbe

17 Fernández, Alexia. 2019. "Hilary Duff Opens Up About Deciding to Stop Breastfeeding After 6 Months: 'I Was Going to Break.'" *People*, May 7. https://people.com/parents/hilary-duff-opens-up-stopping-breastfeeding/

18 Jones, Sarah. 2019. Amy Schumer Reveals Why She Stopped Breastfeeding Her Son: 'This is Not for Me.'" *The Independent*, December 31. https://independent.co.uk/life-style/amy-schumer-breastfeeding-son-gene- formula-pumping-baby-a9265256.html

19 American Academy of Sleep Medicine. 2007. "Baby's Conception and Birth Can Influence Dream Content in New Moms." *ScienceDaily*, September 2. https://sciencedaily.com/releases/2007/09/070901073638.htm.

20 Galoustian, Gisele. 2016. "New Study Looks at 'Love' Hormone and Mother-Infant Bonding." *Florida Atlantic University News Desk*, March 22. https://fau.edu/newsdesk/articles/mother-infant-bonding.php.

21 Gordon, Karen. 2024. "What I Wish I'd Known about Life with a Newborn." *Babycentre UK*, March 12. https://babycentre.co.uk/a1046160/what-i- wish-id-known-about-life-with-a-newborn.

22 Westmaas, Reuben. 2019. "What Would Happen If You Stayed Awake for 11 Days?" Discovery.com, August 1. https://www.discovery.com/science/What-Would-Happen-Stayed-Awake-Days

23 Keating, Sarah. 2018. "The Boy Who Stayed Awake for 11 Days." BBC, January 19. https://bbc.com/future/article/20180118-the-boy-who-stayed-awake-for-11-days

24 Pitman, Teresa. 2018. "Why Babies' Tears Make Us Cry and Why They Matter." *La Leche League International.* November 28. https://llli.org/news/why-babies-tears-make-us-cry-and-why-they-matter/.

25 Ibid.

26 Low, Felicia. 2022. "Perinatal Mental Health in Aotearoa: An Under-Recognised Concern." *Helen Clark Foundation*, September.

https://helenclark.foundation/app/uploads/2022/09/ATR-roundtable-presentation-2-slide-deck-Dr-Felicia-Low.pdf

27 New Zealand Treasury. 2022. *Maternal Mental Health Report 2022.* https://treasury.govt.nz/sites/default/files/2024-05/pc-inq-fcfa-sub-086-maternal-care-action-group-nz.pdf.

28 Ibid.

29 Slomian, J., G. Honvo, P. Emonts, J.-Y. Reginster, and O. Bruyère. 2019. "Consequences of Maternal Postpartum Depression: A Systematic Review of Maternal and Infant Outcomes." *Women's Health* 15. https://doi.org/10.1177/1745506519844044.

30 Paterson, Kristina. 2015. "Postnatal Depression in New Zealand and Feedback on Maternal Mental Health Services." *Mothers Helpers.* https://mothershelpers.co.nz/wp-content/uploads/2015/12/NZ-PND-Survey-Results.pdf.

31 Mothers Helpers. 2019. "How is NZ faring? Mothers Helpers release latest survey." Scoop, May 1. https://scoop.co.nz/stories/GE1905/S00006/how-is-nz-faring-mothers-helpers-release-latest-survey.htm.

32 Parts of this chapter originally appeared as "Nappkin Charity Helps Overwhelmed New Mums." *Stuff*, April 4, 2024. https://stuff.co.nz/wellbeing/350218348/nappkin-charity-helps-overwhelmed-new-mums.

33 Klein, Jessi. 2016. *You'll Grow Out of It.* Grand Central Publishing.

34 DeRoche, Hayley. "daddy made you some new content, thank you for your patience as I've been away being sad." TikTok, September 29, 2022. https://tiktok.com/@sadbeige/video/7148600576996134186

35 Holmes, Marie. 2023. "What Is 'Sad Beige' Parenting, And How Did We Get Here?" *HuffPost,* January 24. https://huffpost.com/entry/sad-beige- parenting-trend_l_63c5cf84e4b0cbfd55f587f3

36 Metcalf, Hugh. 2023. "Is It Actually Okay to Have an All-Neutral Nursery? Here's What a Psychologist Says About the Viral 'Sad Beige Baby' Trend." *Livingetc,* July 30. https://livingetc.com/news/sad-beige-baby.

37 Cosslett, Rhiannon Lucy. 2023. "Why is Mum-Shaming Still a Thing in 2023? Is it Because Society Still Won't Let Women Fully Express Themselves?" *The Guardian,* September 15. https://www.theguardian.com/commentisfree/2023/sep/15/mum-shaming-2023-women-bad-mother.

38 Atkins, Lucy. 2004. "'I Was So Completely Traumatised by the Fact That I Hadn't Given Birth.'" *The Guardian*, March 23. https://theguardian.com/society/2004/mar/23/health.lifeandhealth.

39 Reynolds, Mark. "Why Kated lied about Mia's birth." *Daily Mail.* https://www.dailymail.co.uk/tvshowbiz/article-300032/Why-Kate-lied-Mias-birth.html

40 Children's Commissioner. 2018. "Who Knows What About Me: A Children's Commissioner report into the collection and sharing of children's data." November 8. https://assets.childrenscommissioner.gov.uk/wpuploads/2018/11/cco-who-knows-what-about-me.pdf.

41 Longbottom, Jessica, Carla Hildebrandt, and Dunja Karagic. 2024. "Inside the World of 'Kidfluencers' Where Children Make Thousands from Social Media – At a Cost." *ABC News*, May 21. https://abc.net.au/news/2024-05-21/kidfluencers-children-instagram-social-media-four-corners/103810250.

42 Bath, Gemma. 2024. "Every morning, Zoe deletes messages of men sexualising her daughter." Mamamia, June 18. https://www.mamamia.com.au/child-influencer-risks/

43 Grose, Jessica. 2020. "Fighting Constantly After Baby? Read This." *The New York Times*, May 8. https://nytimes.com/article/fighting-after-baby-guide.html.

44 Eldemire, April. 2016. "Romantic Relationships Take a Dive After Baby Arrives (According to Research)." *The Gottman Institute*, November 18. https://gottman.com/blog/romantic-relationships-take-a-dive-after-baby-arrives-according-to-research/.

45 Johnson, Matthew D. 2016. "Want to Save Your Marriage? Don't Have Kids." *The Guardian*, May 24. https://theguardian.com/commentisfree/2016/may/24/marriage-kids-children-relationship-suffers-research.

46 Schulte, Brigid. 2015. "The Relationship Lessons We Can Learn from Gay Couples." *Stuff*, June 5. https://stuff.co.nz/life-style/love-sex/69150788/the-relationship-lessons-we-can-learn-from-gay-couples.

47 Schulte, Brigid. 2015. "The Relationship Lessons We Can Learn from Gay Couples." *Stuff*, June 5. https://stuff.co.nz/life-style/love-sex/69150788/the-relationship-lessons-we-can-learn-from-gay-couples.

48 Dunn, Jancee. 2017. *How Not to Hate Your Husband After Kids*. Little, Brown and Company.

49 Hogenboom, Melissa. 2021. "The Hidden Load: How 'Thinking of Everything' Holds Mums Back." *BBC*, May 19. https://bbc.com/worklife/article/20210518-the-hidden-load-how-thinking-of-everything-holds-mums-back.

50 Ibid.

51 Miller, Claire Cain. 2018. "A 'Generationally Perpetuated' Pattern: Daughters Do More Chores." *The New York Times,* August 8. https://nytimes.com/2018/08/08/upshot/chores-girls-research-social-science.html.

52 Hogenboom, 2021. "The Hidden Load." *BBC.*

53 Lovell, Chloe. 2021. "Having a Baby Doesn't Have to Mean the End of Your Friendships." *Cosmopolitan*, February 19. https://cosmopolitan.com/uk/reports/a35279220/having-baby-young-friendships

54 Stokes, Rose. 2023. "'I've Been on Both Sides of the Parenting Friendship Divide. This is What I've Learnt'." *Women's Health*, September 15. https://womenshealthmag.com/uk/health/a45136113/parenting-friendship-divide/.

55 Kawther, Alfasi. 2020. "The Loneliness of Early Parenthood." *The Atlantic*, February 5. https://www.theatlantic.com/family/archive/2020/02/loneliness-early-parenthood-mothers-estrange-friendships/606100/

56 Healthify. 2022. "Infertility (Mate matapā)." December 19. https://healthify.nz/health-a-z/i/infertility

57 Powell, Candace. 2022. "How Infertility Can Rip Friendships Apart." *Today*, May 1. https://today.com/parents/pregnancy/infertility-friendships- rcna26130.

58 Stokes, 2023. "'I've Been on Both Sides of the Parenting Friendship Divide. This is What I've Learnt'." *Women's Health.*

59 Jones, Sarah. 2019. "Growing Number of Men Lose Close Friends in the First Year as Fathers." *Independent*, June 10. https://independent.co.uk/life-style/new-fathers-day-friends-lose-baby-support-stress-dads-a8951721.html.

60 RNZ. 2021. "Toni Street's Memoir of Heartbreak and Hope." Interview with Jesse Mulligan on *RNZ Afternoons*. September 28. https://rnz.co.nz/national/programmes/afternoons/audio/2018814155/toni-street-s-memoir-of-heartbreak-and-hope.

61 Zurowska, Aleksandra. 2025. "Global Infertility Rates Rising, Study Finds." *European Medical Journal,* February 22. https://emjreviews.com/reproductive-health/ news/global-infertility-rates-rising-study-finds/.

62 Te Aka Matua o te Ture Law Commission. 2022. *Review of surrogacy.* NZLC R146. April 29. https://lawcom.govt.nz/our-work/review-of-surrogacy/tab/report.

63 Parts of this chapter originally appeared as "Sinead Corcoran Opens Up about Living with Derealisation Disorder." *New Zealand Herald*, October 23, 2022.

64 Dunne, Nathan. 2019. "'I'm Not Me': A Bizarre Disorder Leaves People Feeling Distant from Their Bodies." *The Washington Post,* June 30. https://washingtonpost.com/health/im-not-me-a-bizarre-disorder-leaves-people-feeling- distant-from-their-bodies/2019/06/28/aab4a75e-5d48-11e9-842d-7d3ed7eb3957_story.html.

65 Renfro, Kim. 2021. "Bo Burnham's new special has a lot of people Googling 'derealization'. *Business Insider*, June 8. https://www.businessinsider.com/bo-burnham-inside-derealization-meaning-that-funny-feeling-2021-6.

66 Merz, W. M., R. Fischer-Betz, K. Hellwig, G. Lamprecht, and U. Gembruch. 2022. "Pregnancy and Autoimmune Disease: Diseases of the Nervous System, Connective Tissue, and the Bowel." *Deutsches Arzteblatt International*, 119(9), 145–156. https://doi.org/10.3238/arztebl.m2021.0353.

67 "Ratchet and Clank (characters)," Wikimedia Foundation, last modified 15 May 2025, 18:05, https://en.wikipedia.org/wiki/Ratchet_and_Clank_(characters)

68 Better Business Bureau. https://www.bbb.org/us/ma/boston/profile/online-shopping/temucom-0021-553943

69 Kumar, S. S., A. Rajagopalan, and J. K. Mukkadan. 2016. "Vestibular Stimulation for Stress Management in Students." *Journal of Clinical and Diagnostic Research*, 10 (2), CC27–CC31. https://doi.org/10.7860/JCDR/2016/17607.7299.

70 Lopez, Adriana. 2024. "10 Science-Backed Benefits of Using Sensory Swings." Savoiz, October 16. https://www.savoiz.com/blogs/news/10-science-backed-benefits-of-using-sensory-swings.

71 Jha, Alok. 2013. "Lonely Planet Found Wandering a Mere 80 Light Years from Earth." *The* Guardian, October 10. https://theguardian.com/science/2013/oct/10/lonely-planet-pso-80-light-years-from-earth.

72 David, L. 2015. "Separation-Individuation Theory of Child Development (Mahler)." Learning Theories, December 4. https://learning-theories.com/separation-individuation-theory-of-child-development-mahler.html

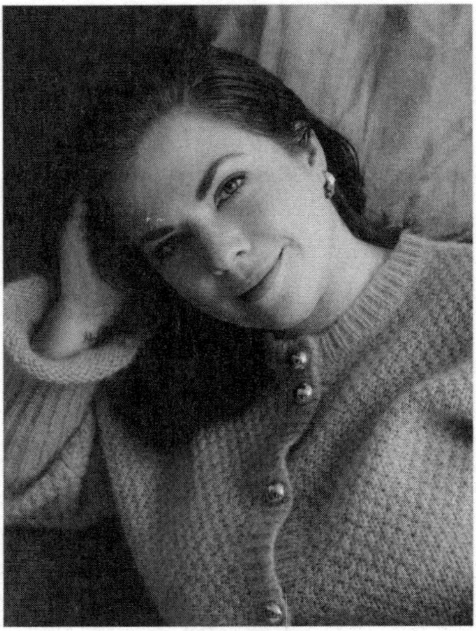

Sinead Corcoran Dye has been a journalist for over a decade, swapping red carpets and the glitz and glamour of her high-flying media career for juggling three kids and documenting the realities of being a young-ish stepmum, a new mum and a working mum. Day-to-day she writes lifestyle and parenting features for *Stuff*, *Canvas*, *NZ Herald*, *Fashion Quarterly* and *Condé Nast Traveler*, and guest stars on local and international podcasts – all while bouncing a baby on her lap. In addition, Sinead is a social media content creator who has amassed a following by being honest about life and love, parenting and mental health. She is the ambassador for Nappkin charity and is the founder of MumSOS, a nationwide community group for mums.